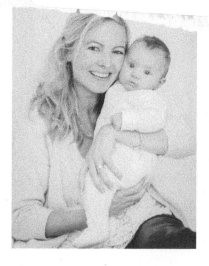

Vanessa Christie (MSc, MN, IBCLC, RHV, RNC, CIMI) is an International Board Certified Lactation Consultant, birth and perinatal trauma practitioner, health visitor, children's nurse, infant massage instructor and a mother of three. She has worked alongside more than 10,000 new families over the past 20 years, predominantly for the NHS and in voluntary roles in South Sudan, Uganda and India.

Vanessa now runs a busy independent practice, The Parent & Baby Clinic, consulting with pre- and postnatal families on a wide range of issues from infant feeding, unsettled babies and sleep, to birth and perinatal trauma recovery.

She is a breastfeeding and early parenting expert speaker for events such as The Baby Show, has contributed to two previous books and writes widely for parenting publications and websites.

VANESSA CHRISTIE

The BABY FEEDING BOOK

Your essential guide to breastfeeding,
bottle-feeding and starting solids
with confidence

piatkus

PIATKUS

First published in Great Britain in 2020 by Piatkus

3 5 7 9 10 8 6 4 2

A CIP catalogue record for this book
is available from the British Library.

ISBN 978-0-349-42387-6

Illustrations © Josephine Dellow
Photographs: p1 © Sarah Legge; p145 top-left © istock; p145
top-right and bottom-left © Jennie Yelverton; p145 bottom-right
© Heather Kemp; p149 © Jennie Yelverton

Typeset in Calluna by M Rules
Printed and bound in Great Britain by
Clays Ltd, Elcograf S.p.A.

Papers used by Piatkus are from well-managed forests
and other responsible sources.

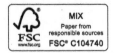

Piatkus
An imprint of
Little, Brown Book Group
Carmelite House
50 Victoria Embankment
London EC4Y 0DZ

An Hachette UK Company
www.hachette.co.uk

www.improvementzone.co.uk

For Amelie, Laria and Eliza

How much do I love you?
All the way to the moon and back a squillion times.

Author's note

This book does not substitute for individual medical, nutritional, psychological or lactation consultations where necessary. Where medication and supplements are suggested as interventions, I have mainly steered clear of stating doses to avoid self-prescribing without seeking further advice and ensuring that this is a safe and appropriate choice for each individual. Please use the Resource section in this book to find further detailed information and always talk to your health professional first.

The language in this book aims to be inclusive of all parents, families and their babies. The author fully acknowledges that not everybody having a baby, and/or producing breast milk for a baby, will identify as female, a mother or a woman. *Any* person can be a breastfeeding or chestfeeding person. For the purposes of continuity and clarity throughout the book, the author uses the terms parent, mother, mum and woman about those persons giving birth and/or lactating, and father, dad and partner when referencing their primary support partner. The author also alternately refers to babies as she and he.

Contents

Introduction

Owning our story and loving ourselves through that process is the bravest thing we'll ever do.

BRENÉ BROWN, PHD, LMSW

Growing up in the 1980s and 90s I didn't consider for a second how I might, one day, feed any potential children of my own. I happily fed my dolls with the bottles they came with and simply assumed that babies always ate gloopy food from a jar. Even at university, training for 4 years to be a children's nurse, I barely thought anything of it. Any mention of breastfeeding was fleeting and never went much further than a brief garble about 'benefits'.

It was only after being set loose on the wards that I started to see things differently. Shift after shift, distraught new parents would turn up with their equally stressed little babies. We'd write on the notes 'crying baby', 'baby not feeding', 'mother has no milk', 'poor feeding' and so on. The standard medical response? Breastfeed every 3 hours (if the mother *was* breastfeeding), top up with formula and observe. With any luck they may have been given a breast pump to try out, which often produced little joy extracting milk (we'll find out why later in the book). The babies guzzled down their formula and were discharged home with 'feeding improved, baby gaining weight' on the discharge letter. Wonderful. But was it?

On the surface they went home chunking up nicely and everyone should have felt happier. But they didn't. The parents were exhausted, physically and emotionally. Often feeling that they'd failed, that they'd let their babies down. They had received next to no assessment on what had been happening and why. We were encouraging them during pregnancy to breastfeed and then, when the proverbial sh*t was hitting the fan, hardly anyone knew how to help. It was cruel.

I went on to do an MSc in Mother and Child Health and realised for the first time that breast milk, breasts and the whole wider process of feeding babies is both a huge and fascinating topic, for all the reasons I share with you in this book. I was hooked. I also realised that as easily as things can go wrong, with the right information and wider social support, things can just as easily go right.

So I set about enrolling myself on more courses, establishing breastfeeding and postnatal support groups, becoming a health visitor, an NHS Infant Feeding Lead, an International Board Certified Lactation Consultant (IBCLC), a practitioner in birth and perinatal trauma recovery, a trained mindfulness practitioner and eventually I established my business, The Parent & Baby Clinic.

I also had two babies of my own. My first baby was 10lbs (4.45kg) at birth. I'm not exactly big (my kids affectionately refer to me as 'the smallest mummy at school') and I found myself on the receiving end of numerous unsolicited and poorly informed comments like 'you won't be able to feed her by yourself' and other equally demotivating remarks from every angle. As it turned out, I could and I did – for 14 proud and happy months.

Fast forward a few years and my second baby was born. Or, for greater accuracy, 'fell out of me', an hour after I woke at home. It was intense and it didn't stop there. She cried. We both cried. A lot. She would take ages to start feeding and once she did, she'd quickly fall asleep and then the whole sorry story would play out again. It was a tough time that slapped me hard in the face when my then 2-year-old asked me one teatime if I could give her 'something I can chew', after days of being served up sloppy microwaveable toddler meals! Aaaargh, the guilt! It took a good 6 weeks and a lot of work and bloody-mindedness before I felt I could breastfeed my baby anywhere other than in a weird contorted position on my bed. We got through it though and I ended up breastfeeding her, alongside food (not all sloppy I might add) for 2 years. I have no doubt that if I didn't have the belief I had that we'd get there, I'd have stopped in those early weeks and would have a different story to tell.

Your feeding book

Once upon a time there were no parenting books. Then one popped up. Then two. Fast-forward to today, there are hundreds, if not thousands. And that's even before hitting Google. So why add this to the mix? Simple. The heady mix of books and websites, together with social media, the experiences of our family and friends and the booming commercialisation of all things baby-related, have

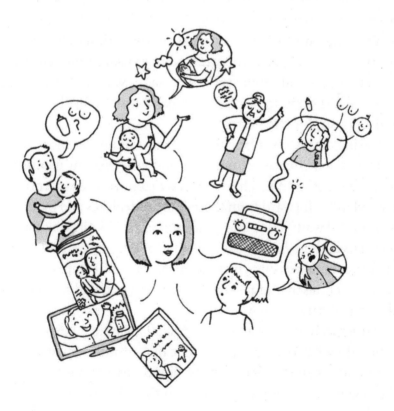

created a whopping great melting pot of direct and subliminal messaging, leading only to confusion for many parents.

The books range from the brilliant to the misleading, but even when you *can* weed out the good information, they rarely account for our individual thoughts and feelings, they frequently sideline (or patronise) any partners and are all too often narrowly focused in their chat, thus missing out on the crucial bigger picture.

I am a firm believer that we can't talk about feeding babies without enough talk about sleep. And we can't talk about feeding *or* sleep without understanding how babies develop and what they can (and can't) do in the first place. All of this should only be given airtime in the first place if flanked with a huge dollop of attention to how we, as parents, perceive and experience the reality of it all. Every parent knows that there is nothing emotionless about having and feeding a baby.

Having worked with more than 10,000 families over the past 20 years, I believe that by being told what we 'should' do with feeding, whilst simultaneously side-stepping all these things, has swollen the tide to tsunami levels of parental frustration, guilt, self-doubt, anxiety, stress and often straight-up sadness on how they judge their own 'success' in feeding their baby. It shouldn't be this way and it doesn't have to be.

Having a baby must be one of the most, if not *the* most, transformative experiences of our lives and every parent deserves to relish and thrive in it. This book is written with the intention to try and move forward from these difficult feelings and big-up the good ones. I want you to know that 'success' looks different for each one of us and can be defined widely by looking at concepts such as greater confidence, enjoyment, connection, self-compassion, self-belief, hope, a sense of personal empowerment, and simply being the type of parent you want to be.

Rather than dictate a one-size-fits-all approach, I explain why babies do what they do. I also offer insight into how it can feel to be a new parent along with the preoccupation with how feeding is going. I explain the whats and the whys of breastfeeding, bottle-feeding and giving solids to your baby in the first year, as well as giving you practical how-tos for your mental and physical toolkit. You can then pick and choose what is right for you and your baby. The book is ultimately about championing your hopes and expectations to help them turn into a reality, giving you the confidence to know that you will be absolutely nailing it in your own way. After all, confidence isn't about looking around and feeling better than everyone else, it's about reducing or eliminating the need to compare yourself to anyone in the first place.

Alongside this, I hope it helps to pave the way for a more holistic and well-informed approach to infant feeding advice, to reduce the misplaced judgement and encourage everyone to have greater compassion for both themselves and others, regardless of differing decisions and circumstances.

We never have the full picture of what is happening in someone's life when we see a snapshot. The mum breastfeeding in the café is likely not there to flash her boobs around and make a statement. She may well have gone through a rough time establishing feeding. She may have been worrying about feeding anywhere outside her home, eventually psyching herself up to get out and give it a go. She deserves a medal. The dad half falling asleep whilst giving a bottle in front of the TV may not be fully engaging with his baby right now because he could have been up all night supporting his partner, changing nappies, drying tears, trying to hold his own back and all whilst getting into work the next day. He deserves a medal too. And the hot-mess of a woman shovelling a shop-bought purée into their crying toddler's mouth, whilst simultaneously flashing a boob on a park bench with a flailing baby ... well, that one was me. I don't know about the medal but what I did need was a reassuring *'this is a crappy moment right now, I get it, and you're doing an amazing job'* smile from a passing stranger.

There are now many networks of professionals and volunteers working tirelessly to improve feeding and postnatal support for families. However, counting the political pennies and the resulting cuts in funding throughout recent years has made taking meaningful strides forward a walk through treacle in most areas of the UK. My wish for this book, written to celebrate and support every family on whatever their feeding journey becomes, is that it goes some way in carrying all this amazing work forward.

Boobs, bottles, bibs and everything in between

This book is meant to be dipped in and out of, depending on what part of the feeding journey you are currently on or need help with. We start with planning how you would like to feed your baby by looking at the evidence, as well as the physical and mental practicalities you may want to consider. We then move through the whole journey of your baby's first year, covering how it can feel to be a new parent and how this is important to feeding. We'll look at how babies are primed to feed and how we can make the most of this, along with practical tips for establishing breastfeeding, bottle-feeding and starting solids. If you have already had your baby when you come to this book, the information in the early chapters will still provide the answers to many questions you may have and give you practical ideas for boosting your confidence in feeding if needs be.

Within the text, there are also different practical facets to the book that you can use as you please, depending what is relevant and resonates with you.

You will find boxes called 'Nikki's zen zones' written by my mindfulness teacher, Nikki Wilson, often with links to free recorded meditations on her website. She says:

As parents, it's normal to have busy brains stuffed full of things we need to do. But when our minds are occupied all the time, we begin to lose touch with the present moment. We get stuck in automatic ways of thinking, mindlessly working down the to-do lists or allowing our own worries and judgemental inner voice to grow louder.

Mindfulness is a counterbalance to this challenge – it's about learning to become more aware of our present moment experience, giving ourselves permission to be still and welcoming what we find with a kind and open heart. When we work in this way we can start to feel a little bit more space between ourselves and our thoughts. Most of us are unknowingly very attached to our thinking patterns and we assume most of our thoughts to be facts. In mindfulness training we teach people that our thoughts are simply mental events of the mind and they don't define who we are or what we are capable of.

The science behind this practice is clear. Negative emotional stimuli, such as anything that provokes fear or worry, can hijack our thoughts by firing off fight or flight signals from an area of the brain known as the 'amygdala'. When the amygdala goes into overdrive it sends our adrenaline soaring and obstructs the ability of the rest of the brain to think clearly. This is intrinsically linked to feeding as you will see throughout the book. Mindfulness practice has been proven to help decrease the extent to which the amygdala flies off the handle and thus allows our rational thoughts to have a louder voice, helping bring about calm and clarity. Whether you are a seasoned meditator or are just stumbling across the idea here, try it out and see how it feels. If it's not your bag, then skip past them.

Secondly, I have written some affirmations at the end of each chapter. The use of positive statements, such as these, has been shown to help question and rise above self-sabotaging and unhelpful thoughts. By repeating them frequently, our thinking patterns can shift, helping us to start believing in what they say and acting as an impetus to make positive change if necessary. Whenever you see one that connects with you, treat it like a hug for your mind. Write it out and keep it somewhere visible or close to hand, repeating it (preferably out loud) as often as you can.

And finally, I have left space for you to clarify and document

your thoughts and plans in the Ponder point boxes throughout the book.

I hope you enjoy *The Baby Feeding Book* and that it leaves you
feeling both confident and calm on your feeding journey.

Vanessa x

1

Your baby feeding planner

Naturally, thoughts during pregnancy tend to centre around how the baby is growing, trying to keep as healthy as possible and making plans for the birth. Yet I would be stinking rich if I had a pound for every time a parent has retrospectively looked back and said to me that they wished they'd *also* delved a little deeper into what feeding was all about, with a view to learning more about their options and feeling more mentally and practically prepared. This chapter will help to do exactly that, by covering all the aspects of getting in the baby feeding zone and building a confident picture of how you see your own plans.

This chapter will explore:

- Components of breast milk and formula milk
- The research picture and grounds on which infant feeding guidance is based
- What breastfeeding means for dads and partners
- If everyone can breastfeed
- Practical planning you may want to consider
- Getting into a positive mind zone and why this is important for breastfeeding

Components of breast milk and formula milk

Being open about breastfeeding and formula-feeding – and the fact that yes, they are indeed different – understandably opens the floodgates of emotion and opinion. What this is not and should never be about is taking so-called 'sides' or guilt-shaming anyone for decisions they may or may not have any control over.

What it *is* about is enabling you, as autonomous parents, to access your right to impartial and evidence-based facts, to help you to develop fully informed thoughts about how you feed your own babies. If you feel that this section may be triggering emotions for any number of reasons, know that I hear you and that you are not on your own. I hope that this book will provide you with the clarity and tools you may be seeking to ease any old or recent hurts.

Formula milk

This is commonly derived from cow's milk and then modified in a factory to make it nutritionally suitable for an infant. It is an inert substance, which means that it comes as it is in the packaging and remains unchanged from one day to the next.

The main ingredients of a standard infant formula are:

- Fats and fatty acids: depending on the brand, these are generally taken from palm, rapeseed, canola, soybean, coconut, sunflower, egg, fish and algal oils
- Carbohydrates: lactose and corn syrup
- Protein: whey and casein from cow's milk
- A wide range of vitamins and minerals: derived from various sources
- Other smaller ingredients: soy lecithin (an emulsifier), a few nucleotides (non-protein nitrogens), free amino acids for supporting growth and development and an enzyme called trypsin, to help digestion of the milk proteins

The ingredients of formula milk is a strictly regulated area and all companies have to meet standard nutritional requirements. Some companies have manufactured additional ingredients that go beyond the minimum requirements, which are commonly marketed as bringing the milk 'closer to breast milk'. These added ingredients have not currently been found, by independent bodies, to be beneficial or necessary for babies and therefore haven't been included in the standard requirements.

For example, some formula milks now market themselves as containing oligosaccharides to 'mimic' Human-Milk Oligosaccharides (HMOs), which are described in the following section. Although it seems a positive step forward for the industry, the impact of adding one or two artificially made oligosaccharides has yet to be proven to make any clinical impression on a baby's health.

Breast milk

This refers to the milk produced by the human body. It is a bioactive, dynamic substance (a bit like blood), which means that it is full of 'living' factors that are ever changing to the environment and the needs of the baby. More is being uncovered about the properties of breast milk all the time.

As things currently stand, breast milk is thought to have:

- Fats and fatty acids: more than 30 human-derived fats, fatty acids and long-chain fatty acids (for optimal brain and eye development).
- Carbohydrates: lactose and more than 200 HMOs (which help to prevent infections and reduce inflammation). The exact composition of these will vary from mother to mother and over the period she is breastfeeding. HMOs are purposefully indigestible for the baby as they serve as prebiotics in the gut. Essentially, they are breakfast, lunch and dinner for healthy gut bacteria and ensure that the baby maintains a healthy intestinal microbiome.

This human microbiome refers to an estimated one hundred trillion microbes (communities of bacteria, fungi and viruses) that live in and on every one of us, predominantly in the gut. This 'super-organ' has a crucial role (many now argue the *most* important role) in maintaining and protecting our long-term health and is therefore vital to keep in balance. Considering that 70 per cent of our human immune system stems from the health of our gut, these microscopic HMOs are truly valuable players in protecting health, not only in infancy but setting up our immune system throughout our lives.

- Proteins: more than one thousand amino acids, proteases, peptides, proteins, cytokines and non-protein nitrogens (for growth, development, immune function and even a specific component called HAMLET which has anti-cancerous actions).
- Vitamins and minerals: as they are made by the human body, these are more readily absorbed by the baby than ones from other sources.
- Millions of anti-microbial and immune cells: this includes many antibodies, live blood cells, stem cells, 'good' bacterial cells and more, to fight infections and reduce inflammation.
- Over forty enzymes: to support the digestive and immune systems.
- More than one thousand microRNAs: these contain the building blocks for gene expression with the ability to help prevent or stop disease progression.
- More than twenty types of hormones: which send messages all over the baby's body to help regulate their emotional responses, growth, appetite and even sleep patterns.
- Fifteen types of sterols: important for cell membrane structure and helps produce vitamins and hormones.
- Lots of water.

Unexpected influences on breast milk composition

Sex. Studies have shown that in general breast milk for boys tends to be slightly higher in fat and protein than breast milk for girls. This is no bad thing as your body knows that boys need to get set up for a little more growing. However, remarkably, in some groups, such as mothers living in severe poverty in Kenya, it has been found to be the other way around and here the girls tend to get higher fat milk. It is theorised that this may be nature's way of ensuring girls survive and produce children.

Age. Once milk production has been fully established by around 2–4 weeks after birth, the volume of milk a mother produces hardly changes at all for the next 5 months, even though the baby will double its birth weight. The composition of the milk itself changes depending on the age and requirements of the baby.

Environment. When a mother is exposed to any potential micro-bial 'threat' such as viral particles in the air from someone else's sneezes, her brain receives a message to produce breast milk with the specific antibodies against that virus.

Health. When a baby is unwell, the numbers of leucocytes (infection-fighting white blood cells) in the breast milk gets a boost. How does the milk know if a baby needs this? There is a strong scientific suggestion that backwash from a baby's mouth is carried into the mother's nipple during a breastfeed, signalling to her body the need to gear up for action.

Time. Breast milk produced at night contains higher levels of nucleotides that relax the central nervous system and promote rest, whilst daytime milk helps to stimulate more activity. It's far from a guarantee of a full night's sleep but every little boost helps!

→

Weather. There's no need for extra water in hot weather as breast milk has it all worked out. When things get steamy, breast milk develops a higher water content to meet the thirst of the baby. Conversely, in cold winter months, it has a higher fat content.

Flavour. As with amniotic fluid during pregnancy, the foods we eat as mothers are passed through in the flavours of breast milk. Exposing babies to all this variety in early life is thought to help their acceptance of food when it's their turn to start.

Toxins in breast milk and formula milk

Occasionally we'll see alarming news stories that report on toxins in the milk we feed our babies. Whilst it would be a lie to claim that breast milk and formula were free from all traces of any toxins, it's crucial to keep this in perspective. In the world we live in today, our exposure to small doses of toxins is everywhere. They're in the soil where our food is grown, in the air we breathe, in the products we have in our homes and in the water we drink. Large studies have found that possible exposure to chemicals in both breast milk and formula are *highly unlikely* to exceed safety guidelines and, in many cases, are seen to be decreasing over time, as both companies and consumers are becoming more aware and starting to use fewer in their homes and in the production of formula and feeding equipment.

Milk testing kits are available on the market, although I strongly advise steering well clear of them. They may entirely unnecessarily create unfounded worry, which is the last thing any new parent needs. Since formula milk is not a toxin-free alternative and because of the *many* ways in which living breast milk works in helping to counteract any potential effects of unwanted elements, it makes sense that if you want to breastfeed, you can confidently go right ahead and do it.

Trusting the research

As we've seen, there is no doubt that the constituents of formula milk and breast milk vary in numerous ways, but what do these physical differences tell us about the impact one way of feeding may have on babies and mothers over another? And should we believe it? We should question the validity of research because not all research is well conducted.

There will always be individual breastfed babies and breastfeeding women who get sick. Likewise, there will always be individual formula-fed babies who seemingly sail through life without so much as having to reach for a paracetamol. These anecdotal examples are wholly valid. On an individual level.

Good quality research digs much deeper than pitching one individual against another and looks at the outcomes across wider groups of people. It also refers to patterns of 'risk' across these population groups. This means that the research does not aim to say that '*all* formula-fed babies *will* get x, y or z' or that '*all* breastfed babies will *never* experience x, y or z'.

In contrast, research explains that when looking across a number of different people, the chance of x, y or z happening is either higher or lower between one group of people when compared to another. In a similar way, no one should suggest that if you wear a seatbelt in a car you will be 100 per cent safe from injury in an accident. There will always be some individuals who are still hurt, even if they were wearing a seatbelt. However, if we don't wear a seatbelt, the overall chance or risk of injury is certainly higher than if we wear one on a regular basis.

But what of the way research is conducted? There are numerous things to consider when looking at research to avoid taking headlines at face value; here are the biggies you should be aware of.

Selection criteria

Although *any* amount of breastfeeding is more than worthwhile, the effects of breastfeeding, in countless research papers, have been shown to be dose-related. That is, the more a baby is breast-fed in infancy and early childhood, the bigger and longer-lasting the effects. If formula is introduced, this will undermine the full effects on the body of exclusive breastfeeding (although in no way makes breastfeeding pointless).

When looking in detail at the methods used in various studies suggesting little difference in outcomes between breastfed and formula-fed babies, it is often clear that the individuals selected for the two population groups can't quite be as neatly categorised as simply having always and only been 'breastfed' or 'formula-fed'.

Babies classified in breastfed categories may have only been breastfed for a very short period of days or weeks, or may have been given a few bottles of formula in the early days. Likewise, the babies in the formula-fed category may well have been breastfed in their earlier life. This type of fuzzy selection criteria waters down the true meaning of the results, since it is well documented that any degree of mixed feeding (that is, a baby having received both breast milk and formula milk) can alter the microbiome, thereby impacting on possible inflammation and immune responses.

Maureen Minchin, renowned researcher and author of *Milk Matters: Infant Feeding and Immune Disorder*, hypothesises that the true impact of breastfeeding is even further underestimated in research because:

- There is very little that accounts for the diet of the mother during pregnancy and how this could impact on a baby's microbiome after birth, and
- That there is likely to be an intergenerational effect on the breast milk we produce today, meaning that

the breast milk produced by a woman who was herself breastfed (and even her mother before that), will be different compared to breast milk she would produce if she was formula-fed (and/or if her mother, the baby's grandmother, was formula-fed).

These effects are part of a much wider area of popular current research into what is 'epigenetics'. This refers to the ability of external factors to modify our genetic DNA by being able to turn certain genes on or off. The influence of these factors (including stress, environmental exposures, diet and how we're fed and cared for as babies, among many others) and their subsequent ability to modify how genes are expressed, significantly impacts on our life-time health and wellbeing. The influence of this gene expression is then carried on through modifications of our genes down the generations.

Recall bias

Another common issue in how research is conducted is recall bias. This relies on parents or other participants looking back and remembering (or not) what may or may not have happened or been observed in the past, with regards to the outcome being measured for the study. For example, parents may be asked to remember whether their child had a chest infection as a baby and the results depend on the accuracy of this recall or not.

Confounding factors

A confounding factor can be anything that could be influential and potentially make the results useless, unless they are considered in the methodology of the research. For instance, two common con-founding factors that come up in infant feeding research are the mother's education level and smoking status in the home. Feeding method aside, both points have been shown to independently impact on a baby's health and wellbeing and should therefore always be fully factored into the research.

Where's the money trail?

It sounds cynical, but it is worth noting that a not-insignificant proportion of research in this area has connections, either through direct funding or by using affiliated researchers, to the formula milk and baby food industry. In an industry currently worth around $40 billion (projected to rise to $70 billion over the next few years) the influence is heavy and the desire to produce research that boosts sales is high on the agenda. It's business after all.

The grounds for the guidance

Since 2003, the World Health Organization (WHO) has recommended that babies are exclusively breastfed (meaning no food or other type of milk) for their first 6 months of life, to achieve 'optimal growth, development and health' regardless of where they live in the world and what access they have to clean water. Thereafter, the guidance suggests that babies should continue to be breastfed, alongside solid foods, up to the age of 2 years or beyond.

How did they draw these conclusions and why stick to them now? As with research about anything, the 'gold standard' for drawing the most reliable conclusions is to look at what are known as 'randomised controlled trials', systematic reviews and peer-reviewed studies. Although I have heavily researched these areas for this book, I am not noting the specifics throughout, for if I started, we'd be going down a deep hole into textbook territory. If you want to investigate any of this further, please do have a look at the Resources (page 285) where you can find links that will guide you to original research papers.

There has been an explosion in the numbers of well-regarded research papers that have been published (and continue to be) in independent medical, immunological, nursing, child development, lactation and psychological publications over the last few decades, which further investigate the impacts of infant feeding. It is these studies that formed the original basis of, and continue to underpin, the official guidelines on feeding young babies.

Their conclusions show patterns across population groups that formula-feeding (to reiterate: this does *not* by any means imply *all* formula-fed babies would be affected) is associated with an increased prevalence of the following issues when compared with breastfed babies (particularly those who are exclusively breastfed):

- Respiratory infections such as pneumonia, bronchiolitis and other respiratory viruses
- Middle-ear infections (otitis media)
- Urinary tract infections
- Necrotising Enterocolitis (NEC)
- Type 1 diabetes
- Gastro-intestinal infections such as diarrhoea and vomiting
- Obesity
- Childhood leukaemia and other cancers
- Sudden infant death syndrome (SIDS)
- Lower IQ scores
- Allergic conditions such as atopic dermatitis, asthma and cow's milk protein allergy
- Some autoimmune conditions and metabolic disorders

Other studies, looking into the impact of infant feeding on the health of women, show distinct patterns (again, across populations) between mothers who have breastfed and those who have not. Their conclusions tell us that to a greater or lesser extent, not breastfeeding presents an overall higher chance of the following:

- Heavier postnatal bleeding and thus an increased chance of anaemia

- An earlier return of periods
- Taking longer to return to pre-pregnancy weight
- Osteoporosis and hip fracture (in the long-term)
- Pre-menopausal breast cancer
- Ovarian and endometrial cancers
- General inflammation increasing the chance of developing autoimmune conditions such as rheumatoid arthritis or diabetes
- Postnatal depression*

A report commissioned by UNICEF UK in 2012, investigating the potential financial contribution of breastfeeding, estimated that even modest increases in breastfeeding rates in the UK would save the NHS around £40 million per year in GP visits and hospitalisations – and this was only looking at a small handful of the conditions above where breastfeeding is thought to have the greatest impact. They felt that the true cost savings were likely to be much more significant.

Breastfeeding after babies get teeth

You may hear people say that breastfeeding is unnecessary or weird after they start to get teeth (which commonly starts at around 6 months). This is often a reason given for wanting to end breastfeeding. The truth is that not one teensy part of breast-feeding a baby or toddler after they get teeth is weird. Conversely it is exactly what a baby biologically expects – human milk made specifically for humans! If it wasn't meant to happen our bodies would know to shut up the milk shop at 6 months and there would be something else to meet their needs that didn't have to be made in a factory.

Once a baby starts eating foods, breastfeeding continues to

---

* If breastfeeding is not going well, this may potentially fuel the development of postnatal depression (see page 47).

give them most of their necessary nutritional requirements well into the second year. In addition, it carries on doing all the things it has always done for protecting and strengthening their immune system and providing comfort and stability for their speedily growing brains and bodies, for as long as breastfeeding continues.

You may hear people tutting about a link between breast-feeding and tooth decay. It was once thought by some that since breast milk tastes sweet it must cause rotting teeth. This theory has been totally de-bunked and research has now found that breastfeeding until at least 12 months actually works as a protective factor *against* tooth decay. Where breastfed babies and toddlers have experienced tooth decay, it is due to irregular and unsupervised tooth brushing. This is a problem because it is known that food left around the teeth (particularly carbohy-drates), in the presence of milk, will help bacteria to ferment and increase the chances of tooth decay. Therefore, regular and supervised teeth brushing from the moment teeth start to erupt from the gums is important, regardless of breast or formula-feeding.

Reasons other than 'health benefits' that motivate many mums to breastfeed

Health reasons aside, many women feel motivated to breastfeed for a range of additional reasons, such as finances, logistics or wanting to lessen their carbon footprint of having kids.

The act of breastfeeding itself is also a powerful parenting tool for physiologically calming both mother and baby and providing a wonderfully deep source of security, connection and comfort. Very often the greatest reason of all is that a mother simply feels a strong instinctual drive to want to do so and because she enjoys it!

I wasn't sure I wanted to breastfeed at all and thought I really wouldn't like it ... Once I gave birth everything changed and I was suddenly desperate to be able to breastfeed her and not to have to bottle-feed. I had this amazing pull to feed her myself.

Bethany

It was about finances for me ... and ease. Not having to pack anything other than breast pads and a muslin cloth. Not having to get out of bed to make bottles. Not having to do loads of bottle cleaning and sterilising. Breastfeeding makes life simpler (in my opinion) and for me means less stress.

Becki

I just wanted to ... I love the skin-to-skin, cuddle time and the sudden rush of relaxation! Now that I have experienced both breastfeeding and using bottles, I love the convenience of breastfeeding. Logistically, especially at night, it's so much easier.

Hannah

Breast milk isn't just for drinking!

Here are some weird and wonderful anecdotal ways parents have made the most of the anti-infective and moisturising goodies in any extra breast milk.

1. Make it into a one-of-a-kind soap with some lavender
2. Whip up a face cream
3. Apply it to stretch marks to help fading
4. Soak like Cleopatra in a milk-bath
5. Use it as an all-in-one first aid kit for cuts, sticky eyes, nappy rash and stuffy noses

Ponder point

Write down what is motivating you, if you are thinking about breastfeeding.

Keeping these thoughts close by and referring to them if times get tricky can help you assess whether or not they are still important to you and why. If they are, these words can help to give you a boost to get the answers and the support you need to help things get easier.

Know who to trust

One thing that comes up time and again for parents is trying to figure out whose advice to trust. It can be a very frustrating and confusing time being faced with lots of different opinions. It is especially upsetting if you feel coerced into following advice that doesn't feel right for you (which of course you don't have to do). Knowing how to weed out sources of dodgy advice and finding informed, objective and compassionate support that holds on to what *you* want at its heart, is often crucial to success.

The most knowledgeable people to speak to at times of need are certified breastfeeding counsellors, La Leche League (LLL) leaders (who often work for voluntary organisations) or an International Board Certified Lactation Consultant (IBCLC), who can all help you with concerns around breastfeeding and bottle-feeding.

Be cautious of self-named 'experts' with little or no specialist qualifications. Unfortunately, the terms 'breastfeeding consultant', 'baby feeding specialist', 'breastfeeding expert' and 'infant feeding specialist', among others, are meaningless terms that do not reflect any specific breastfeeding or infant feeding-related qualification. They may well be kind and understanding people (and some are very knowledgeable) but many will have no actual breastfeeding qualification. In the UK anyone can use a range of titles and seemingly charge a lot of money, confusing families who think they are seeing a true specialist. After all, no one would do a few hours of training in a garage and then call themselves a mechanical engineer!

One place to avoid getting breastfeeding advice is from an industry-sponsored 'careline'. This is nothing against formula as a product, or the likely lovely women on the end of the phone. But there is no doubting that the true goal of these advice lines is to warm parents to the brand and ultimately encourage them to buy their products. I tested this out for myself by ringing up four different lines posing as a mother in distress with worries from milk supply to cracked nipples. Without exception, having been offered some unhelpful advice, I was asked if I wanted them to mail out information on their milks 'just in case'. So there's the answer – honestly it really was nothing more than sugar-coated marketing, to put doubt in my belly and gain my personal information.

Navigating this minefield of where to go for help is tricky for the uninitiated. Hopefully the following table will clarify things; and remember that you are always within your rights to ask someone what their specific related qualifications are.

Position and NHS/Private	Breastfeeding-specific qualification	Breastfeeding education	Breastfeeding experience
Obstetrician, paediatrician, general practitioner (GP) NHS/Private	None required for these positions Some with special interest do additional training and/or may be part of the growing GPIFN (GP Infant Feeding Network) or HIFN (Hospital Infant Feeding Network) in the UK	Minimal exposure in training No mandatory post-qualification training	Generally limited (unless personal experience or a special interest)
Midwife/health visitor/nurse NHS/Private	No statutory requirement for these positions Some take a specialist interest in breastfeeding and will have completed their own further training e.g. as an IBCLC or breastfeeding counsellor (see below)	May have completed a 2–3 day UNICEF Baby-Friendly breastfeeding training course and attend regular updates Others will have also attended further trainings, relevant conferences etc.	Variable

Position and NHS/Private	Breastfeeding-specific qualification	Breastfeeding education	Breastfeeding experience
Dietician/ nutritionist NHS/Private	None required for these positions, although, as above, some have a separate breastfeeding-related qualification	Very limited exposure in training Study days often sponsored by formula companies	Likely to be very limited (may have personal experience or have taken a special interest)
Maternity/ breastfeeding support worker NHS (on maternity wards and in community midwifery teams)	None required for this position	As per midwives/ health visitors/ nurses	Variable
Maternity nurse (Note: This is a non-medical term referring to nannies who look after families with newborn babies in the home) Private	None required for employment	Some may have completed an MNT (maternity nurse training) course which typically consists of between 2–7 hours of training on breastfeeding May also have a special interest and attended further courses	Variable

Position and NHS/Private	Breastfeeding-specific qualification	Breastfeeding education	Breastfeeding experience
International board certified lactation consultant (IBCLC) NHS/Private/Voluntary	IBCLC is the only internationally recognised professional breastfeeding qualification The examining body is IBLCE	There are different pathways to become an IBCLC. Most candidates are health professionals or have a recognised BF support counsellor qualification. They then complete a minimum of 90 hours of recent BF-related education prior to sitting IBCLC exam IBCLCs are required to complete on-going education after qualifying and re-certify every 5 years	Health professionals and BF counsellors/LLL leaders (see below) are required to have a *minimum* of 1,000 hours' recent experience in BF counselling prior to being eligible to sitting the IBCLC exam Many IBCLCs have thousands of hours' experience with breastfeeding families

Position and NHS/Private	Breastfeeding-specific qualification	Breastfeeding education	Breastfeeding experience
Certified breastfeeding counsellor, breastfeeding supporter or La Leche League leader NHS/Private/Voluntary	Accreditation awarded in the UK by organisations such as the NCT, ABM, BfN and LLLGB. Some have university accreditation	Average 2 years part-time Continuing education requirements vary between organisations	Variable For most organisations, they must have breastfed their own baby for a significant time prior to training
Voluntary breastfeeding peer (or mother-to-mother) supporter NHS/Voluntary	Awarded by individual organisations or trusts	Average training of 16–36 hours Continuing education should be offered	Variable Usually mothers who have breastfed themselves
'Breastfeeding specialist', 'breastfeeding consultant', 'baby feeding expert' (these are not protected titles) Private	None required	No pre-requisite May have completed short breastfeeding training mornings/days. Some may be maternity nurses (see above)	Variable

Ponder point

Search online for breastfeeding resources local to you. Note down the names and contact details of drop-in groups and individuals below so that you have them to hand if needs be.

Breastfeeding and bonding for fathers, partners and other family members

It's a common worry that breastfeeding automatically means that anyone other than the mother could struggle to bond with the baby.

If you are the one breastfeeding, there should be no pressure whatsoever on you to let someone else 'have a go' at feeding, if this is not what you want or need to do. It is very much a personal choice. Some mothers relish the opportunity to hand over the reins, whilst for others it just feels like extra work having to express instead. If feeds at the breast are missed, this inevitably leads to soreness and a drop in milk supply – particularly in the early months. When you've put in all the initial effort to get things going, it can feel very undermining to be made to feel guilty or selfish for not giving this up and introducing a bottle.

What's the alternative? First off, remember that breastfeeding itself is the *only* thing that you can't do as a father, partner, grandparent, friend or anyone else involved with the mother and baby. There really are countless other ways to bond with the baby, whilst also being an amazing source of support to the mother.

Here are a few practical ideas to get started:

- **Do bath-time.** Or even better, get in the bath with your baby. There is nothing weird about it. This is a wonderful opportunity to help a baby relax, have lots of skin and eye contact and have a giggle too.
- **Settle the baby after a feed.** Cuddles, shushing, rocking, patting or even a bit of salsa dancing (whatever floats your boat) can very much be in somebody else's domain, as and when Mama is having time out.
- **Skin-to-skin snuggles.** This isn't just the preserve of mothers. There are many benefits for having a cuddle with the baby stripped down to a nappy and their father or significant other taking their top off or down. Wrap a dressing gown or blanket safely over the top of you both and soak up the love. One word of caution though – never fall asleep whilst a baby is on your chest, as this can be extremely dangerous.
- **Changing nappies and dressing.** It may sound boring but these opportunities actually provide a fantastic opening to interact with a baby. Singing, stroking, tickling, whispering, smiling, eye contact, funny faces and silly voices, are all the building blocks of not only a positive relationship between the two of you, but will also help their fast-developing brains to learn positive communication, love and empathy.
- **Take the baby for a walk.** For extra bonding time and super-cute daddy brownie points, try out a soft baby carrier.
- **Give the baby a massage.** The benefits of massaging babies are bountiful and have been proven to increase

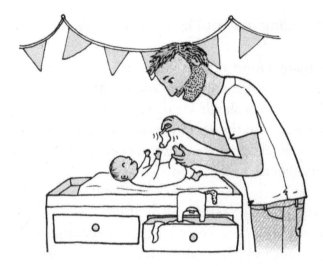

the release of hormones, in both the baby and carer, that
help promote bonding and loving behaviour. Look into
finding a baby massage course near you, or if you don't
have any going on, there are a wealth of online videos
that can show you the way.

- **Sing songs and read.** Babies are sensory beings and they
love hearing familiar voices. It doesn't matter if you
think you sound silly or are reading total gibberish. It
will be heaven for your baby and every time they hear the
sound of your voice it will draw them closer to you.

*My partner's done nappy changes, bath-time, cuddles/skin-to-
skin, singing, stories, playing, everything!*

Bobby

*I do occasionally express now so he can feed the youngest
but I didn't with the eldest and there's no difference to their
relationship.*

Yazmin

Breastfeeding may not be for everyone

Whilst many issues can be prevented or overcome with good information and perhaps some additional professional support, not *everyone* can or should breastfeed fully or at all. The statistics vary depending on the definitions used, but this is generally considered to be relevant for under 5 per cent of mothers and babies in situations such as the below.

- **Mothers taking certain medications**

Most medications are compatible with breastfeeding since, in general, only tiny and insignificant amounts make it through into the breast milk. Some of the main cases which are contraindicated include chemotherapy medications, iodine, lithium (*may* be possible with strict monitoring), gold salts and retinoids.

A few other medications require a baby to be monitored for signs of side-effects (such as some psychiatric and anti-convulsant drugs), or using alternative drugs could be suggested in other cases (such as certain antibiotics and decongestants). If you are unsure about any advice you have been given regarding your medications and their compatibility with breastfeeding, check out the Resources section (page 285).

- **Mothers who have a condition such as:**
  - Active herpes simplex virus type 1 (with lesions on the breast)
  - Active breast cancer treatment
  - Active tuberculosis (TB)
  - HIV*

---

* HIV is a particularly complex one. In the developed world where access to safe water and formula are readily available, it is currently advised that mothers who are HIV Positive do not breastfeed, although anti-retroviral medication virtually eliminates the risk of transmission via breast milk if a baby is being exclusively breastfed (mixed feeding is known to increase the chance of transmission). However, in developing countries, where the weight of risks and benefits can be very different, the advice for mothers is commonly the opposite and exclusive breastfeeding is often recommended.

- Untreated brucellosis
- Syphilis lesions on the breast or nipple
- Having had a double mastectomy

- **Some metabolic conditions in the baby**

On very few occasions an unwell baby may be diagnosed with a rare metabolic condition shortly after birth, such as maple syrup urine disease (MSUD), phenylketonuria (PKU) or galactosaemia. Breastfeeding babies with MSUD and PKU should not be a total no-no. However, the amount of breast milk these babies receive will be closely monitored so that they do not ingest too much of certain amino acids which are problematic to their condition. Any shortfall in the amount of breast milk that is safe for them to drink is then made up with specialist formula milks.

Galactosaemia is generally regarded as fully incompatible with breastfeeding. Once these babies have been diagnosed they will be prescribed a lactose-free formula that is safe for them to drink.

Red flags that *could* make producing breast milk more of a challenge

During pregnancy, many women experience tender breasts which tend to get bigger, particularly during the first trimester. This is a comforting sign that the body is getting prepared and things are all as they should be. However, for a small proportion of women, the process of making breast milk doesn't kick-start itself quite so efficiently. There are some pre-determined circumstances when breastfeeding is certainly possible but could be more challenging and requires some specialist help.

- **Previous chest or breast surgery**

Many women who have had surgery to their chest or breasts are able to fully breastfeed their babies without supply issues, even where a mother has had a single mastectomy. Breast reduction surgery tends to have the most significant impact on milk production, although any other type of breast, chest or nipple surgery may also influence the process, due to possible disruptions to important nerve supplies and/or milk ducts. How much supply is affected will depend on the type and location of the surgery, as well as how long ago the surgery was performed. As for nipple piercings, most mothers will be able to breastfeed without any complications, especially if the piercing was done at least a few years prior to having a baby. However, there is a possibility that some piercings may lead to a chance of blocked ducts and mastitis. If relevant, be sure to remove any piercings prior to feeding to avoid a possible choking risk and damage to the baby's mouth.

- Hormonal disruptions

The process of making breast milk involves a fair few hormones. Anything that puts a possible kink in their chain, such as a history of cranial radiotherapy as a child, polycystic ovary syndrome (PCOS), diabetes, thyroid abnormalities or hormone-related fertility difficulties, could *sometimes* make things more challenging but it is certainly more than feasible in most cases.

- Mammary hypoplasia, also referred to as insufficient glandular tissue (IGT)

These hormonal disruptions can occasionally lead to a condition where the breast(s) did not fully develop the expected amount of glandular tissue (the milk making parts) during puberty or pregnancy. There is also some research to indicate that genetic factors and long-term exposure to various toxins, such as pesticides or chemicals in domestic products, can also influence this process. Affected breasts may have a marked tubular shape, lop-sided appearance and/or sit widely spaced on the chest. Confusingly, they can also sometimes appear full and round where there may be additional fatty tissue, despite glandular tissue being on the low side.

- High body mass index (BMI)

If you have a high BMI of 35 or above and are keen to breastfeed, then don't let this be a worry to stop you forging ahead. If the will and determination are there, you are already several rungs up the ladder to success. Some women with a high BMI do find that building and sustaining a full milk supply is a challenge, and there are emerging theories that this may be related to the complex interplay of various hormones, including leptin and prolactin, and the effect they have on milk production.

Other factors

The following factors could lead to breast milk being slow to appear or cause longer-term milk supply issues (if unchecked):

- Low stimulation of the breasts by the baby (and/or an expressing pump) due to poor advice on positioning the baby at the breast, a baby who is struggling to latch on, introducing a strict feeding schedule or early introduction of formula milk.
- Feeling acutely stressed or exhausted.
- Certain aspects of labour and birth that *may* affect how ready a baby is to feed after delivery (including induction with synthetic oxytocin, or instrumental deliveries such as the use of forceps or ventouse) and opiote-based pain relief medications.
- Excessive intravenous (IV) fluids pre-birth can lead to swollen breasts and make it hard for the baby to latch and stimulate the breasts.
- A large blood loss or incomplete delivery of the placenta, affecting the hormones necessary for milk production and possible development of anaemia.
- Preterm birth (as breast growth in pregnancy is cut short), but with optimal breastfeeding management, breast development will continue after the birth of the baby.

If any of this should ever turn out to be relevant to you, know that help and resources are available and things *will* become better and easier. If you are worried, speak to a breastfeeding specialist such as an IBCLC, who will be able to chat through this with you. Find information on different ways of maximising milk supply if necessary starting on page 167.

Breastfeeding with an autoimmune condition

In themselves, conditions such as systemic lupus erythematosus (SLE), multiple sclerosis (MS), rheumatoid arthritis (RA) or inflammatory bowel disease (IBD) are not necessarily a contraindication to breastfeed, although each mother should seek individual advice. In most cases breastfeeding has not been found to be a primary exacerbating factor in potential postnatal flare-ups (except for some women with RA and particularly with a first baby). There is no chance that breastfeeding will pass on the condition to the baby and, on the contrary, some researchers firmly believe that breastfeeding is a protective factor for reducing the overall chance of a baby developing various autoimmune conditions in their later life.

The main considerations for families tend to centre around medication, fatigue and general wellbeing. Most medication prescribed for autoimmune conditions is compatible with breastfeeding, although this should always be checked out. Often drug companies will advise caution because little is known about any long-term effects. If your doctor says 'no' outright, then do research this further as there are common misconceptions about what is safe or not in this area. Go to Medications and breastfeeding advice and information on page 286 for further resources.

With fatigue and wellbeing, this is a very personal decision that only you can make, depending on your own feelings and circumstances. Whilst some women find that breastfeeding works out to have a lower labour intensity, is easier to manage physically and is very enjoyable for them, others may feel that a combination of breast and bottle-feeding, or fully bottle-feeding, is the right path and easier for them. This book contains many tips and tricks to help minimise fatigue and the general 'work' of breast and/or bottle-feeding your baby.

Worries about saggy boobs

It's a widespread worry that breastfeeding will lead to saggy boobs. The truth is that it isn't breastfeeding itself that does the job, it's simply the hormones and changes involved in being pregnant in the first place. Other contributing factors are smoking, genetics, age, BMI and overall muscle tone. So whether you breastfeed or not, it's likely that your breasts will look just the same at the end of the day.

The diversity of our breastfeeding and bottle-feeding journeys

Infant feeding can be far more diverse than simply being in a straight 'breastfeeding' or 'bottle-feeding' camp. There are an assortment of ways to feed your baby if you aren't able, or wish, to exclusively breastfeed, depending on the individual needs, wishes and resources of your family.

Without formula options
- Exclusive breastfeeding
- Breastfeeding + expressed breast milk (EBM)
- Breastfeeding + EBM + donor breast milk

With formula options
- Breastfeeding + EBM + formula
- Breastfeeding + formula
- EBM + formula (with no direct breastfeeding)

- Exclusive donor breast milk (with or without 'dry' breastfeeding where a baby suckles for comfort but is not accessing any milk)
- EBM + donor breast milk
- Formula + 'dry' breastfeeding
- Formula + donor breast milk
- Exclusive formula

If none of this breastfeeding talk sits right with you

You may be reading all this feeling that formula-feeding sits more comfortably with you. Your thoughts may include:

- It will give my family and me more physical freedom
- The family can join in with the feeding
- I tried breastfeeding before and it didn't work
- I'm worried that it just won't work for me
- I need to look after older children as well
- I don't know anyone who has breastfed or enjoyed it
- I don't want to be restricted in how I eat, drink or exercise
- My partner doesn't want me to
- I want to get into a routine and I've heard it's harder to do with breastfeeding
- I have to go back to my work, education or training soon after the birth
- I just don't like the thought of breastfeeding

Any concerns and thoughts that you have are real to you and therefore entirely valid. You may find that after reading through the information in this book your perspective alters and you may feel reassured that breastfeeding, for some or even all the time, could well feel right for you after all. Or not! And that's

OK! Without question you are in control and absolutely have the right to say no to anything you don't feel comfortable with. Making decisions on how you feed your own baby are for you and only you to make. If you're not sure how you feel or what you want to do, always know that no plans or decisions ever must be fixed in advance. You could simply start with some skin-to-skin cuddles after birth and see what may or may not lead on from there.

Practical planning before your baby arrives

When it comes to planning the practicalities of how breastfeeding could fit with your personal circumstances, your body and your lifestyle, here are some things you may want to consider during pregnancy.

Tandem breastfeeding

Breastfeeding through pregnancy is more than possible and many more women than you may think are doing exactly this. Our bodies are truly incredible at figuring out what needs to happen, and gradually during pregnancy the milk adjusts itself and reverts to colostrum ready for the new baby. Some older babies and toddlers will wean themselves from the breast as this is happening, only to sometimes start wanting to breastfeed again later, once they get wind of what their baby brother or sister is up to. The main thing to remember is that the new baby gets priority at the milk bar to ensure they are getting what they need.

Breastfeeding without having been pregnant yourself

Breastfeeding without having been pregnant is possible and can be a powerful way to physically and emotionally connect with your baby. This may be relevant to parents expecting their baby

through surrogacy or adoption and members of the LGBTQIA*
community, such as transgender parents and those in a single-
sex relationship, where both parents would like to be able to feed
their baby (known as 'co-nursing'). Increasing numbers of people
around the world have prepared their bodies to induce lactation
(the process of producing breast milk) for these reasons and have
gone on to breastfeed (or chestfeed) their babies either partially or
even fully for many months.

The protocols for inducing lactation and the outcomes do vary,
depending on how much time there is before the baby is due to
arrive with the family, how old the parent is, how developed the
breast glandular tissue is (this is particularly relevant for tran-
swomen) and what they feel comfortable doing. Generally, the
process of making breast milk in these circumstances involves
a combination, adjusting over a period of time, of birth control
pills, the medication domperidone, herbal supplements and breast
stimulation through hand massage and breast expression.

Flat or inverted nipples

Breastfeeding with flat or inverted nipples is certainly possible
although it may take a little pre-planning and some additional
support to get things on track. If your nipples persistently stay
at the same level as your areolae (the darker circle around your
nipple) regardless of stimulation, or if they seem pulled back
beneath the level of your skin, the odds are that you have flat or
inverted nipples.

It may be hard to tell just from looking so you can try the pinch
test – position your hand with your thumb and forefinger in a C-
shape, placing them an inch behind the nipple on either side of the
areola, gently push your thumb and finger in towards your ribcage.
A common nipple will move forward, a flat nipple will remain
unchanged and an inverted nipple may retract into the breast.

---

* Lesbian, Gay, Bisexual, Transgender, Queer or Questioning, Intersex and Asexual.

Don't panic if either of these things are happening. During pregnancy the breasts do gain elasticity and the fibrous adhesions which hold the nipples back often loosen naturally. It's also vital to remember that babies breastfeed and don't nipplefeed, which means that they latch on to the area around your nipple and not the nipple itself. They use the nipple purely as a guide to get them to the right place.

Nevertheless, when these guides aren't standing up for duty, it's useful to seek some specialist support to help you optimise how to hold and latch your baby and ensure that your milk is being removed from your breasts well enough to prevent engorgement, which can flatten and aggravate things further.

There are various gadgets on the market that purport to draw flat and inverted nipples out through gentle suction. These get mixed anecdotal reports, most likely depending on how elastic the individual's nipple is. There is no independent research that suggests they make a significant difference although you may wish to give them a go and experiment. A manual technique that uses thumb pressure to supposedly encourage adhesions to release is known as the 'Hoffman Technique' and has been around since the mid-twentieth century. To carry this out you put your two thumbs on either side of your nipple, apply gentle pressure into your breast and then stretch your thumbs away from each other. You then continue to do this all around the nipple. This can be done for a couple of minutes a few times each day. Again, whilst there are many mothers who report to have used it to good effect, there is little controlled scientific evidence that it works.

Colostrum harvesting

Colostrum (the first milk) starts being made in the breast from around 16–22 weeks of pregnancy and you may want to do some occasional hand expressing to collect and store some in the freezer, from around 36–37 weeks. Having a few syringes of colostrum at the ready (which can quickly defrost) for when your baby is born, can put your mind at ease if, for any reason, you are separated, unable to breastfeed immediately after birth or your baby needs a little extra milk to help stabilise their blood-sugar levels in the early days.

Colostrum harvesting can also be particularly helpful if you have:

- Diabetes
- Gestational diabetes
- A raised BMI
- A baby with cleft lip or palate
- A twin or other multiple pregnancy
- A baby with Down's Syndrome
- A baby who is small for their gestational age

What's more, physically seeing that you have milk there ready and waiting will undoubtedly be a reassuring boost to your confidence.

Since we are talking about tiny drops of milk here (don't expect torrents!), the most efficient and effective method to collect the colostrum is simply by using your hand – you can ask your midwife how to do this. Your midwife should provide you with a syringe pack and show you how to do this during a one-to-one appointment, or possibly at free antenatal group sessions that are available in some areas. If nothing seems to be forthcoming, just ask. If it doesn't seem to be working, don't panic. It has no reflection on your ability to make milk once your baby is here.

Placental encapsulation

This is the practice of having the placenta dried and made into capsules for mums to take in the weeks after giving birth. There are many advocates who believe that it boosts iron levels in women, promotes positive mental health and can increase breast milk supply, with plenty of anecdotal stories available in support of these claims. From a scientific point of view, the evidence remains mixed and solid conclusions simply aren't available yet. Looking specifically at milk supply, some researchers and theorists believe that this practice may have a *negative* impact on the production of milk, due to the possible effects of the hormonal levels in the capsules. All in all, it's a confusing picture at present. However, it can be said with certainty that as toxicity levels in the capsules appear to be very low, they are deemed as safe to take.

Practical planning for after your baby is born

Nutrition

The average breastfeeding mother who eats enough to maintain a steady and healthy weight will require roughly 300–500 extra calories per day. This is roughly equivalent to a bowl of porridge, a banana and a piece of toast. If you have a current or historical eating disorder and calorie intake is challenging, it is understandable to feel anxious about this. Try to be honest with your midwife or health visitor, who will listen without judgement and offer you any additional support you may need.

As for what to eat, there are no specific restrictions that need to be followed in order to provide nutritious breast milk. If your life isn't about quinoa, curly kale and carrot juice, your milk will still be gold label, although keep in mind that sugar and junk foods won't do any favours for your sluggish energy levels and low moods. If your diet is plant-based, you can be reassured that you are getting everything both you and your baby need by eating daily good sources of protein, choline and zinc and taking supplements, particularly vitamin B12, vitamin D and iodine.

It's worth noting though that whilst eating a tonne of high fat foods will not make any difference to the *amount* of fat in breast milk, there is strong evidence to show that the *type* of fats we eat (particularly during the last trimester of pregnancy) does have an influence on the *type* of fats in our breast milk. So, this is a great time to get fishy with your diet to boost DHA* levels (useful for brain development of your little one and even influences their mood and mental health in the long-term). If you'd prefer a plant-based source of DHA opt for algae products.

Babies born to mothers with enough levels of vitamin D generally have a liver packed full of vitamin D stores and will get some additional vitamin D in breast milk and from sunlight. However, being sure of getting enough exposure to sunlight (for both mother and baby) in the Northern Hemisphere and eating enough from the limited amount that is available in food is tough. Since 2016, all breastfeeding mothers and breastfed babies from birth to one year old, are advised to take a vitamin D supplement. If you know that your iron levels are dwindling a little in pregnancy, taking an iron supplement will ensure that your baby is born with sufficient stores (boosted by waiting until the umbilical cord has stopped pulsating before it is clamped, known as 'delayed cord clamping'), together with the iron in breast milk, to happily see them through at least the first 6 months of life. Once your baby is born, the iron content of your breast milk will not be affected by your iron count or by taking supplements.

Some people believe that it's important to drink milk to make 'good' breast milk. This is untrue. During pregnancy, the calcium requirements your body absorbs from your gut doubles, however during breastfeeding it returns to normal. If you need to increase your calcium intake, this is for your benefit only as calcium levels in breast milk are not affected by your diet. Your body will use calcium that is already laid down in your bones and calcium supplements have little to no impact on this process. Don't worry about your bone health though, as studies show that bone mineral density returns to normal levels within 6–12 months of birth and may even go back to levels *higher* than they were previously.

---

* DHA (Docosahexaenoic acid) is a type of omega-3 fat which supports brain function and eye health. It is also associated with heart health and with reducing inflammatory responses.

Alcohol

The short answer is yes, you can have an alcoholic drink and feel entirely guilt-free about it! However, there are a few T&Cs to make sure it's safe and appropriate for both you and the baby. It's ideal to stick with around 1–2 units, once or twice a week. The best time to have a drink is towards the end of a feed as the alcohol takes around 30 minutes to 1 hour to peak in your milk. As with caffeine, this will still be in minimal amounts and it takes approximately 2 hours in total to clear 1 unit out of the milk. Therefore, feeding just before having a drink or towards the end of a feed will give you the longest possible time until your baby feeds again. If you're caught out *on occasion* and your baby wants feeding earlier than you expected, don't worry, it will still be safe to feed them.

Binge drinking is a slightly different ball game, so if you've had a splurge it's best to wait long enough until you feel completely sober before breastfeeding your baby. 'Pumping and dumping' will not get rid of the alcohol in your breastmilk (only time does this), although you may need to express purely for your own comfort in your breasts. If you know you'll be having a lot to drink, expressing in advance so that your baby can continue to drink your milk is useful.

Two further points worth noting are:

- Regular binge-drinking could impact negatively on milk supply
- *Never* sleep with your baby in the same bed if you or a partner have been drinking

Caffeine

When caffeine levels are at their peak in breast milk (around 1–2 hours after ingestion), they are still only tiny compared to that in the mother's blood circulation. In spite of this, caffeine takes at least 2–3 days to clear out of a newborn's system, compared with only a few hours for a 6-month-old, so it is possible for some new babies to be sensitive to caffeine building up in their bodies. It is thought that having around 200mg of caffeine in 24 hours is a reasonable limit. This equates to roughly two mugs of tea or coffee (instant or filter) or around five cans of Diet Coke per day (not that I'm suggesting that's a great idea!). Signs of caffeine-related stimulation in a baby include increased wakefulness or fussiness. If you think this may be going on, it may well be worth ditching or minimising caffeine for a few days to see if this makes any difference.

Smoking

If you do smoke you can still breastfeed. There are even constituents of breast milk which help lessen some of the effects of passive smoking on the health and development of a baby. Nonetheless, smoking can negatively impact your letdown reflex (the process of shifting the milk out of your breast), which can lead to issues with frustrated babies not getting all the milk they need. It is also important to note that even if you are breastfeeding, smoking is well documented to have marked health effects on a baby, such as breathing problems, ear infections, behaviour difficulties and increasing the risk of sudden infant death syndrome (SIDS).

If you smoke as a breastfeeding mother, try to aim to have a cigarette immediately after a feed, so that the level of nicotine in your breast milk is at its lowest by your next feed. If you would like to stop but are finding it hard, ask your midwife, health visitor or GP for information on local stop smoking services. Nicotine replacement therapies such as gums, patches, lozenges and sprays are safe to use whilst breastfeeding. Although e-cigarettes and vapes are safer than smoking, they are not entirely free from risk as they do still contain nicotine and toxic chemicals.

Recreational drug use

Breastfeeding after taking drugs such as cocaine and cannabis isn't recommended. Cocaine rapidly makes its way into breast milk, potentially making babies very irritable and causing them to develop a tremor, vomiting and diarrhoea. There is also research pointing to regular use of cannabis affecting a baby's nervous system and delaying motor development. It's suggested to wait for a minimum of 24–36 hours after taking cocaine or cannabis before breastfeeding again.

Beauty procedures

As the research is currently very limited, most practitioners will advise against having botox or fillers during the period a baby is being breastfed. The chance of harm is limited but, as it comes with a question mark, it's better to play safe. Beauty procedures believed to do no harm to a breastfed baby include hair dying and tooth whitening.

Feeding out and about

This is an easy one from a practical standpoint. In the UK you can feed *wherever you like*. If you have a legal right to be there yourself, then you have a legal right to breastfeed there. And that's pretty much most places. What's more complex is how you might feel about it in the first place from *your* personal point of view. Does it faze you to see other women breastfeed? Whatever you feel, it's useful to reflect on where our feelings stem from. Often, it's simply because we're not used to seeing breastfeeding in our daily lives and, when adding in the sexualisation of breasts in everyday western culture, it's little wonder that we might feel awkward about it at the outset. If you are considering breastfeeding but feel uncomfortable about this side of things, following some of the ideas later in this chapter for fostering a confident mindset could make a huge difference. There are also plenty of thoughts on page 178 to help relieve any apprehension you may have.

Getting back to work, education or training

With a little planning, there is no reason why being in this situation need hinder your breastfeeding plans if you don't want it to. Whilst more and more companies are getting up to speed with family-friendly policies and flexible working, every company in the UK should respect workplace regulations that require the provision of 'suitable facilities where pregnant and breastfeeding mothers can rest'. The Health and Safety Executive (HSE) advises employers that their policies should include providing a suitable space for women to express and store breast milk, which does not mean being directed to the toilets! You will find information from page 217 about how expressing for when you are separated from your baby could work for you.

Being of 'advanced maternal age'

Anything age-related you may have heard about the breast milk of older mothers not being of 'good quality' or that age directly affects milk supply is unfounded gibberish. It is known that as we age our metabolism starts to slow down, which *could* leave some women feeling more tired. In an indirect way, tiredness could then increase acute stress, which may reduce milk supply. This can be avoided by listening to your body and doing whatever you need to do to try and ensure you feel as rested as possible.

Caring for older children

The thought of breastfeeding with any other children to look after is a natural worry for some parents who may feel that they will have their hands too full to breastfeed. Yet there are also scores of women who joke that they are 'too lazy' to bottle-feed and find it far less hassle to whip their boob out and get on with it, rather than having to bother with the work of bottles.

As the early weeks pass by, feedings do tend to become quicker overall and, as each mother and baby become more familiar with what they're doing, it's not uncommon for mothers to suddenly start to find themselves feeding one-handed on the floor, sitting next to the bath whilst the toddler splashes about, or opening the door to the postman and all other sorts of multi-tasking!

Breastfeeding evidently means that the baby spends plenty of time physically close with their mother, which could invoke feelings of jealousy and upset in a small child who is used to having all the attention. I remember thinking in my foggy postnatal days that the whole idea of having another baby was a total mistake because I couldn't handle seeing my eldest daughter getting upset. I assure you that this does pass. Here are some ideas to help minimise worries and acclimatise them to this new normal.

- Explain in age-appropriate language what the baby is doing and why. Role-playing this with your child will help them to understand too.
- Help them feel important and valued by asking them to do little jobs (depending on their age), such as finding nappies, helping you to lift your top, gently stroking the baby's back and so on.
- Carry the baby in a sling/soft carrier between some feeds so that you have your hands free to engage with other children.
- Set up a 'feeding time toy box' with some surprises and things they have chosen, which are activities you can do together on the sofa, at the table or on the floor during feeds (e.g. puzzles, drawing, stickers, books, threading, Lego & small imaginary play figures).
- Aim to work in 10–15 minutes each day (once it's feasible) when you can have one-to-one time with them. If your child is physically affectionate and/or enjoys rough and tumble play, try to use this time to have as much physical contact as possible. This will help them feel 'topped up' and hopefully relieve some of their need for this at other

times, which could be harder to accommodate with the baby around.

And finally, the finances

Having a baby can be eye-wateringly expensive if you really want it to be. Got a cool £10,000,000, yes £10 million, to spend on a solid gold cot? Go right ahead, they exist! On the flipside, things don't have to get too expensive at all, including when it comes to feeding.

Formula-feeding

Milk
As explained earlier in the chapter, all milks must conform to statutory regulations governing their ingredients. This means that the cheaper milks are on a par with the more expensive milks. Fully formula-fed babies roughly get through around 6 900g tins of milk per month in the first 6 months and 3–6 900g tins monthly from 6–12 months, slowly reducing as their intake decreases.

Bottles
You'll likely get through 20–30 bottles and teats in the first year. If you choose glass baby bottles these will last longer.

Sterilising system
The cheaper options are cold water sterilising or a basic microwavable steam steriliser with the electrical steam sterilisers being more expensive.

Bottle brushes
It's important to be able to clean bottles and teats thoroughly.

There are a plethora of non-essential but possibly useful bottle-feeding products available on the market:

- Insulated bottle carriers
- Bottle warmers
- Powder dispensers
- An insulated flask
- A feeding pillow

Electric formula preparation machines are also available to buy. These machines are not currently recommended by the NHS or medical professionals. Find out more in Chapter 6.

Breastfeeding

Women have been breastfeeding across cultures for millions of years and of course have managed to avoid trips to the shops. However, we live in different times and the baby product market is booming, meaning that you could find yourself spending more than you anticipated on various, often unnecessary, paraphernalia. Remember that many of the items listed below could be borrowed or bought second-hand (if you need them at all), further saving money and being kinder to the planet at the same time.

Breastfeeding bras

Your breasts will most likely change size again so don't splash too much cash antenatally just in case they don't fit after the birth (and poorly fitting bras can be a risk for mastitis). Like with any bras, there are grim ones out there but also numerous pretty and practical ones. Some also now come with flexible and gentle wire support, designed to move with your changing shape and thereby minimising the risk of causing blockages in your milk ducts. It's best to avoid these for the first few months and women who are prone to mastitis or blocked ducts should steer clear completely. Keep the night shift in mind and invest in a few comfy night bras, to have support in bed and a means to keep any breast pads in place.

Breastfeeding-friendly clothes

Whilst there are loads of brands now creating tops, dresses and jumpers for feeding, you don't have to spend much, or any money on them if you don't want to. With my own kids I tended to rotate a couple of breastfeeding vests with the clips on the straps and then put any of my regular clothes on over the top. That way I could lift my normal top up, unclip the vest and away we went.

Breast pads

These are thin, absorbent pads to wear inside your bra to soak up any leaking milk and protect your clothes. Some women get through boxes of them and others find they never need one. This has no reflection on your overall ability to make enough milk for your baby, so don't panic if you find you're not using them. Disposable breast pads are some of the many things that end up in landfill. An antidote to this issue is investing in a few washable breast pads, which tend to be made from organic bamboo or cotton flannel and are super-soft.

Breastfeeding pillow

By no means an essential part of breastfeeding, you may find you never need one at all, at least not beyond the first week or two. Pillows can become more of a hindrance than a help, although in the very early days when you are tired, achy and getting used to holding your baby, you may well feel that it provides you with a little comfort. If you can, borrow one from a friend, or just use a normal one from home. Some form of pillow or cushion can be especially useful if you have twins or have had a Caesarean birth and have a tender scar to look after. With time and practice, feeding will get much easier and you won't need the extra hassle of carrying a pillow about.

Nipple cream

In the early weeks applying a nipple cream to keep the area well moisturised can help with potential soreness. The most common ingredient in these creams is lanolin, a natural moisturiser derived from shorn sheep wool. It works a treat for many, although it can occasionally cause an itchy reaction in a few women. Other options include creams that are vegan-friendly and contain ingredients such as vitamin E, vitamin A, calendula, coconut oil and shea butter. Breast milk itself does a great job too and is free!

Expressing device

Expressing is not an essential or even necessary part of breast-feeding if your baby is feeding well and you are happy with the way things are. Unless you know that you will definitely need one early on (e.g. you have to be away from your baby for any reason) I would urge you to hold off spending on one during pregnancy. Many hospitals, community teams and breastfeeding groups have pump rental schemes where you can access hospital-grade pumps (the best in the biz) either for free or at minimal cost if expressing becomes necessary. If you are going to get anything at all, cheap silicone breast pumps can be super-handy in the early days, as an alternative to hand expressing for colostrum or to ease any engorgement.

Onesie

A onesie is the perfect way for you to stay warm and keep your baby safe at the same time, whilst lying in bed and feeding on chillier nights.

Feeding tech

Living in the times we do, it's not a surprise to find that technology has made it into the world of breastfeeding. Products that are definitely *not* recommended by breastfeeding organisations, or anyone who understands how breastfeeding works, include those that claim to measure how much milk a baby is swallowing (believe me, these are far from accurate and can be either falsely reassuring or anxiety-provoking) and testing kits apparently measuring the 'quality' of breast milk (again, this is completely off-the-wall as breast milk changes throughout every feed, hour by hour and day by day).

There are also a wide variety of feeding apps now available for both breast and bottle-feeding, to track how often a baby is feeding, what breast they were last on, how much was in the bottle and so on. The use of these apps essentially comes down to the user's personality type and whether it helps induce a sense of calm and control, or if it is just one more thing to have to think about, and therefore unduly increases stress.

Getting in the breastfeeding mindset

As well as figuring out the practicalities of breastfeeding, giving some thought to how you feel about breastfeeding yourself can genuinely help to make a breastfeeding plan turn out the way you may hope.

Consider how you felt when you learnt to ride a bike or the last time you took an exam. Do you remember falling off your bike and thinking 'sod it, this isn't for me'? Or turning over the exam paper and deciding within moments that you were doomed for a meeting in the Head's office with your parents? Or would you say that you were the kind of kid who was fairly bloody-minded and stuck with the bike until you cracked it, or looked at the exam paper and thought 'this is tough but I'm going to make the best job of it I can'?

This mindset, or way of thinking, is largely driven by self-efficacy, which is the innate belief we have in ourselves to accomplish tasks or goals. Self-efficacy is affected by several factors including personal experience, our observations, the influences and support networks around us and also physiological cues from our own bodies, such as sweating and how we breathe.

I have no doubt that this is immensely relevant when it comes to breastfeeding, where there is clearly a strong interplay between how we feel about our ability to breastfeed (plus mothering in general) and how it is physically playing out. For example:

YOUR BABY FEEDING PLANNER   47

- Feeling good in ourselves, confident with our feeding decisions and happy about how breastfeeding is going, is likely to increase its longevity and enjoyment.
- Likewise, even if breastfeeding isn't going so well, where we still have a confident mindset we are likely to have greater resilience, be more prone to seek out support, take better care of ourselves (resting, good nutrition and so on) and ride through tough times to reach outcomes that we are happy about.
- When our anxiety levels are higher but find that breastfeeding is in fact going well, anti-inflammatory effects in the brain (through the activation of the oxytocin system whilst breastfeeding, covered in the next chapter) helps us feel more confident, positive and has been shown to reduce the risk of postnatal depression.
- However, if our anxiety is high, self-efficacy is low AND breastfeeding is not going so well, this can lead to much self-doubt, a sense of powerlessness, exhaustion and guilt. These feelings can override the anti-inflammatory effects of any breastfeeding that is happening and our stress system (comprised of adrenaline and cortisol) is likely to be activated instead, thus increasing the likelihood of stopping breastfeeding before we'd originally wanted to.

Preparing the mind for breastfeeding is ultimately about getting to a place where you feel confident in knowing what it is you'd like to do, whilst having a little perspective on the realities of how things may or may not play out. This can help develop greater self-efficacy and thus a growth mindset, where we believe more strongly that things can adapt and develop. If you decide that you want to breastfeed, remembering how and why you made that decision and seeing things with a forward-thinking 'growth' mind can really help to maintain optimism and see you through possible tougher times.

An example of a fixed breastfeeding mindset may look like this:

Everyone in my family has struggled with breastfeeding, so I know that it isn't going to work for me either.

Or, conversely . . .

Everyone in my family has found breastfeeding easy and I know I will love every minute.

Ironically, even though both women have totally different thoughts, the chances are high that with such a fixed mindset, both women may struggle (mentally and/or physically) at some stage in the game.

Let's look at these two examples again but now considering a growth mindset:

Everyone in my family has struggled with breastfeeding. I am going to try and understand why it was hard for them and then make plans to see how things can be different for me.

Or . . .

I am confident that breastfeeding is going to work with my baby and I am also prepared to ask for help to see me through any challenges that I'm aware may crop up, without beating myself up about it.

I believe that having, or working to develop, this growth mindset, is *the* number one tool to nurture as an individual or as a couple. It could help you to get to where you really want to be, both physically and emotionally, in respect to how you feed your baby.

Practical ideas for building a growth mindset for breastfeeding

For most parents, the furthest they will get in terms of 'preparing' for breastfeeding during pregnancy is attending an antenatal breastfeeding class and buying a bra or two. This is a great start. If you want to dig a little deeper, there are more simple ways that you can build up the breastfeeding scaffolding, so that if the building (i.e. you!) starts to get a little crumbly, you already have a pre-built frame of strength around you. I have seen many times how this can and will go miles in helping you to have both an easier time feeding and to feel more confident and calm in times of need. Here are a few ideas that may work for you.

- **Start by brainstorming any thoughts, words or feelings you have about breastfeeding.** Anything at all that comes to mind. Once you have put it all down, take a moment to think about where these have come from. Perhaps after reading this book, come back to them and challenge them. Are they accurate? Are they a true representation of reality?

- **Address any existing breastfeeding experiences which may have been negative or even traumatic.** This could include having seen a friend or family member in distress whilst feeding their baby, reading difficult breastfeeding stories online, or having a personal experience breastfeeding a previous baby that has left you feeling concerned about how things will go this time around. You may want to 'get it all out' by writing down everything and anything relevant or confiding in a trusted friend whom you know will listen without judgement and simply let you speak. If you feel that you need professional input, arranging a one-to-one session with a certified breastfeeding specialist, to enable you to find some clarity on what may have happened and why with any previous babies, can be hugely beneficial. Having a session with an understanding practitioner certified in gentle fear release techniques can also offer a swift and safe method for shifting negative thought patterns towards a calmer and more confident viewpoint.

Nikki's Zen Zone

Seeing thoughts as just thoughts
A nice Zen exercise to appreciate that 'thoughts are just thoughts' is to stand at the window or take yourself outside. Look up at the sky and observe the clouds for a short while. Clouds gently drift and change with every passing moment, just like the thoughts in our mind. If it's dark outside, just imagine a tree with birds on the branches. Birds sit there a while before moving on and flying away to the next destination – just like your wild and precious mind.
   Go to: www.100fzen.com/awareness and listen to 'Breathe and Come Back'.

- **Address any other worries you have about any specific personal circumstances** in an antenatal session with a certified breastfeeding specialist. As a few examples, if you have a disability, a personal history of abuse or if you know that your baby is likely to have additional needs, seeing a lactation consultant prior to the birth is very likely to help you feel more confident in your thoughts and plans.
  Get visual. One of our major barriers to feeling confident in our own ability to breastfeed comes down to the fact that it's not necessarily something that we see everyday in the UK. When we don't see something happening that often, if at all, it naturally seems a little alien and daunting.
     There are easy ways to counter this and it's never too early or too late to start:

  - Get on to YouTube and you will find fantastic breastfeeding videos (OK and yes the weirdo bitty ones too but stick to the normal ones).

- Follow breastfeeding influencers and hashtags on Instagram, such as #normalisebreastfeeding, #breastfeedingsupport, #breastfeedingmama and #breastfeedingbaby for tons of inspiring and often funny pictures and stories of real-life breastfeeding.
- Visit a local breastfeeding drop-in group. These may be run by your local midwifery or health visiting teams in a children's centre or by a charity or local voluntary-funded group in cafés or churches. Most people there will have already had their baby but you will always be welcome to attend antenatally as well.
- Design yourself a breastfeeding vision board. I know it sounds kooky but trust me, they help! Having a breastfeeding Pinterest board is one thing but it's even better to have a hardcopy vision board that you can put up somewhere on the wall at home, somewhere you are going to see it at least a few times a day. Cut out any positive and inspiring words and pictures you find from magazines, the internet or leaflets and add to it with any of your own creative sparkle too.

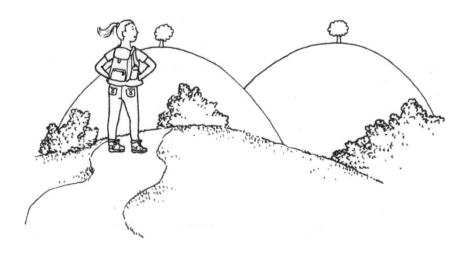

- **Start to apply these visual pictures and ideas to yourself.**
  After a few weeks of following these previous ideas,
  you may well be surprised by how your ideas of seeing
  yourself breastfeeding are changing. Now is a great time
  to start personalising these images and create a picture
  of what it looks like for YOU to breastfeed:

  - Visualise your own breastfeeding experience by closing
    your eyes, becoming conscious of your breath and
    using your imagination to take yourself to a place that
    you find deeply relaxing. Your happy place. It may be
    somewhere you have been or simply a place your mind
    creates. Once there, take a moment to create a picture
    in your head of you calmly and happily breastfeeding.
  - Repeating positive breastfeeding and postnatal
    affirmations out loud to yourself may not be up
    everyone's street but if you have done something
    like this before, or are willing to give it a go, I can't
    overstate how powerful they can be. Use the ones at
    the end of each chapter as a starting point, or, if you
    prefer, make up your own.

- **Build a breastfeeding 'village'.** Whilst it's often said
  that 'it takes a village to raise a child', I am a strong
  believer that it also takes a village to raise a parent. We
  were never set up to do this alone and the evidence is
  indisputable that women breastfeed more happily and
  for longer when they feel they have a solid supportive
  network that has their back.
  Depending on your situation, this 'village' may be ready
  and waiting for you, or it may take a little work to start
  to build the foundations. So where to start?

  - Your own family and existing friends. In an ideal
    world they live close by, are rooting for you, will listen

closely to what is important to you and want to help in any way they can. We all know that life isn't always this straightforward and I've discussed coping with any resistance you may possibly face a little later.

- Make new friends. Whether it's through a 'dating' App for new parents or simply diving in and starting up conversation on the street, connecting to like-minded new parents can lead to all sorts of awesomeness.
- If you have a partner, spend a little time sharing your thoughts about what you both envisage feeding your baby will look like.
  - What are you both excited about?
  - What are you both feeling nervous or worried about?
  - How do you see things working out?
  - How long would you like to breastfeed?
  - What are your roles going to be?
- Having a little clarity about where you both are with your thoughts will undoubtedly help to reduce any unexpected conflict when your baby is born.
- Find local feeding support. Write down and keep somewhere close to hand the contact details of your local support groups, breastfeeding professionals, helplines and online closed support groups (such as moderated Facebook groups).

Ponder point

List at least four things that float your boat from the ideas above (or your own) that you can aim to do yourself.

How to handle opposing opinions about your feeding choices

Most people want the best for each other but, even where there's a lot of love, there remains plenty of potential for debate. As Nikki says:

> All parents are yearning for certainty, looking for ways to make the right decisions which will meet their child's needs. Usually when we feel like we've found something which works, we tell ourselves that it was because we made the best decision and often deep down the decision other parents should make too. So we share these with others hoping for unsung recognition and validity. Conflict arises when we don't feel this validity or if other opinions jar with our own search for certainty.

Regardless of whether you are someone who bats off challenging comments without hesitation, or worries very much about what other people think, it never feels good and can quietly sow seeds of doubt in even the hardiest of hearts. Some clichés never get too old and so I will say it here and you can repeat it to yourself a thousand times:

It is YOUR baby and YOUR body.

No one else has an inherent right to tell you what to do, or not to do, with your body and your baby.* If you are a couple, it is essential to keep lines of communication as open and as calm as possible. Listen to each other and find out what each other needs.

---

* The only exception being in cases where a parent is putting themselves and/or their baby (intentionally or not) in a situation that has the potential to cause, or is causing, significant harm.

Nikki's Zen Zone

Managing conflicting opinions
The world can feel packed full of different views but when it comes to parenting, this fact unites us all – we're all searching for what's best and doing the best we can.

Pause for a moment and expand your awareness into the community of people surrounding you. Imagine all the fellow parents, where everything feels new and uncertain. Like you, they wish to be happy, free from doubt and difficulty. You can imagine sending them some kind vibes or simply say 'may you be as happy and healthy as it is possible for you to be'. Come back into the room when you're ready.

Go to: www.100fzen.com/kindness and listen to 'Classic Kindness'.

My husband fully supported any decisions I made as he saw them as best for my daughter and for myself. That made it easier to ignore other people's 'helpful opinions'.

Constance

I had a lot of negative comments from health professionals that I was bottle-feeding and at that point, with my first child, these were unhelpful. I grew a thicker skin with my second child.

Ellen

I think my family was hesitant about breastfeeding because it was very foreign to them and they just wanted me to do what they saw as 'easiest' and would cause me the least stress.

Helen

AFFIRMATIONS

- I trust myself to make decisions that feel right for me and my baby
- I am not afraid to ask for help if I need it
- I move forwards free from fear
- I do not compare myself to others

2

Settling into life as a new parent

The cards and texts say, 'enjoy your blissful baby bubble' and 'soak up every moment as it goes so fast'. It's true. To a point. Parts of it are blissful and in the long run it does fly by, but I'd be lying if I said it is always going to be a rosy walk in the park. This chapter focuses on everything you are or could go through as a new parent, including:

- Changes that occur in our brains when we become parents and why some degree of heightened awareness and low-level anxious thought is to be expected.
- The power of oxytocin to maximise the feel-good factor; why this is connected to feeding and many practical ways to encourage our brains to flow with the good stuff.
- Recognising how more pronounced mental health challenges, such as significant anxiety, postnatal depression or trauma might present themselves and what to do if you are worried about this.

That first moment of holding your very own baby in your arms is a unique and incomparable experience. There may be an intense 'flood of love' when the most powerful protective instincts, total joy and absolute wonderment about what's just happened kick in. Or at this moment and for some time after, the overwhelming thoughts and feelings may be entirely alien to the former scenario. It could bring up unexpected feelings and confusion. There may be sadness if you are unable to share this time with someone you love dearly. There may be shock and numbness if your birth experience was far from how you'd pictured it. There may be fright and guilt if you are separated from your baby for reasons out of your control. There may be sudden fear and panic about whether you feel 'up to the job'.

If this is you, know that you are not alone and that these are normal reactions to experiences that couldn't be further from our conventional pre-baby daily life. Know that feelings of love will come, albeit sometimes with a little time, and be patient with yourself.

What has all this got to do with feeding? Absolutely everything. How we feel about feeding our babies and how we then travel down those often twisting paths is intrinsically built in to how we feel in ourselves and see ourselves as new parents. This is a good thing if it's working positively in our favour but not so great if it's not.

Blooming brains

Becoming a parent doesn't happen in the flick of a switch the minute the cord is cut. It's a process, an evolution. It's a period which requires self-compassion and patience because no one really knows what the hell they're doing on day one. Or even on day 1001.

As with adolescence, we don't suddenly hit 13 and know how to 'adult'. I have strong memories of needing to buy a new carpet at home after an unfortunate incident at age 14 involving a drinks cabinet and my stomach; kissing far too many boys at 15 and subsequently being off school for 4 months with glandular fever; getting in a dodgy unofficial taxi at 17 and narrowly avoiding the leery driver's advances; and disappearing off everyone's radar in southern India for weeks at a time aged 18, only to wonder why on earth my parents may have been concerned.

Much like these dodgy times, becoming a parent is a time of continuous learning where we grow from mistakes. This period of tremendous physical and emotional change in both women and men is defined by the terms *matrescence* and *patrescence*.

The process kicks off for women when the maternal wiring of the brain starts to change with the flood of hormones in pregnancy, during childbirth and then breastfeeding. It dials up the grey matter in the brain, key to nurturing and being 'on alert' for the new baby. So we're not just blooming on the outside, but inside too!

Physical brain changes are not just confined to women. Dr Anna Machin, evolutionary anthropologist, broadcaster and author of *The Life of Dad*, has studied fatherhood for the past 12 years. She explained to me how men are biologically primed to father:

When a man becomes a father for the first time his testosterone drops and it never returns to pre-fatherhood levels. This makes sure that the man's focus is shifted from finding a mate, to caring for his new family. We also know that the lower a man's testosterone the more sensitive a parent he is and the more motivated he is to care for his baby. Some men are a bit concerned about the drop in testosterone as we associate it so closely with masculinity but the lower your testosterone the more of a positive kick you get from the dopamine and oxytocin which are released when interacting with your baby, so in return you get the most amazing reward and a strong bond. We also see changes in the actual architecture of the brain. Mirroring what happens in a new mum we see increases in grey and white matter in the areas of the brain linked to care and nurturing, these sit at the centre of the brain in the limbic system and increases in the neocortex where our conscious mind sits. Here the increases are in areas linked to problem solving and planning, both key parenting skills.

The degree to which these changes happen in both sexes varies from person to person. Even though researchers are still working on determining exactly what factors mediate the level of change, we now know that we're not simply imagining it when we feel different in how we're thinking and feeling.

The 'dialling up' in our brains helps us to survive from day to day with dramatically altered sleep patterns and ensures that even in the toughest of times parents kick ass at ensuring that their babies are safe and not abandoned. However, there is a snag: anxiety and high emotion.

It's thought that between 50–80 per cent of women will go through some 'baby blues' days in the first week or two after having a baby, often peaking at around days 3–5. It doesn't mean you're losing your mind. You have just had a baby! Feeling overwhelmed, crying over just about everything, struggling to fall asleep (regardless of what your baby is up to) and being snappy and irritable are all very common symptoms of the blues. Despite all this, the predominant mood is happiness and the baby blues often go as quickly as they arrived.

Nonetheless, increased anxious thought continues to linger for many new parents. Although the degree to which these affect how we function varies hugely. On one level, being on high alert is not only normal but valuable and reflects how much a parent loves and cares. However, if it is causing continual racing thoughts and worries, an inability to sit still, shortness of breath and/or heart palpitations, seek some support.

> With my first daughter I was fairly anxious about everything. Any little hiccup or cough had me Googling. It didn't really help. Following my gut instinct turned out to be the best thing I could've done.
>
> **Jessica**

> There were days I felt I was failing and as the baby had colic, the afternoons were particularly challenging. I would cry as much as him. The first few months are a joy but hard and it's OK to admit it's not all wonderful.
>
> **Lesley**

I worried about everything and looking back realise that babies are pretty resilient. You obviously can't be daft about safety, but they're more OK than you think they are ... The internet rarely helped! You can find the negative diagnoses to anything within seconds and in the middle of the night this is very unhealthy. If I have a second baby, I'll know that every stage passes in a heartbeat and that something that's a problem in that moment or week, will change soon enough. This too shall pass is my mantra.

Laura

Nikki's Zen Zone

The big emotions of parenthood

Often as new parents we become intimately acquainted with our emotions and discover the full breadth of our emotional range. The spectrum swings from deep love and joy at one end, to the tougher stuff at the other such as guilt, anger, fear, anxiety and exhaustion. Our ability to yo-yo, without warning, from one end of the scale to the other, often comes as a shock.

Societally, we're not taught that all these feelings are normal, real and valid responses to parenting. We fall into the easy trap of believing that experiencing uncomfortable emotions means we're failing in some way. When really all it proves is that we're human. Emotions have passed through millions of years of human evolution to tell us something. Sometimes the message serves us, at other times it does not. We can be much kinder to ourselves by accepting that it is *real to feel*, remembering that our big emotions demonstrate how much we care.

Whenever any of these big emotions are bubbling, try taking three deep and purposeful breaths – focusing on a nice long exhale if you can. Then lift one hand and place it over your heart centre and simply ask yourself 'what's here for me right now?'. You can name the emotions coming up for you if it helps, such

→

as 'tired', 'nervous' or 'tearful'. Then try offering yourself some comforting words like 'it's real to feel', 'it matters that I care' and 'it's OK'.

Go to: www.10ofzen.com/emotions and listen to 'It's Real to Feel'.

The power of oxytocin

The link between feeding difficulties, anxiety, stress and exhaustion is a catch-22. When any one of these kicks off, it's amazing how quickly they fuel each other. How then is the cycle broken, with the best possible outcomes for both you and your baby?

The good news is that the answer is already inside us. The brain has thought this one through: oxytocin.

Oxytocin is a hormone and neurotransmitter with skills. Without oxytocin in our bodies we'd be emotionless grumps. We'd struggle to feel loved or give out any love, since it fuels those feelings of connection and warmth and it's even been implicated in the intensity of an orgasm. No one would be able to give birth spontaneously, as it is key for getting the contractions going, or subsequently to breastfeed, since oxytocin rules the letdown reflex to make the milk shift out of the breast to the source.

The flipside of oxytocin is that it can also turn us into raging animals when we sense threat to our babies. I'll never forget my unsuspecting husband taking our firstborn out for a walk when she was about 3 weeks old, leaving me at home to have a sleep. I tried and failed. Then the longer I lay awake, the more I stressed out. I started pacing about. Where the hell were they? About 2 hours passed by. I called his phone repetitively. My boobs were bursting and I was on the verge of calling the police. Then he came home. A blissed-out dad with a snoozing baby in the carrier. I. Lost. The. Plot. Cue *seemingly* irrational and uncharacteristic arguing and tears. It turns out though there was science behind it after all. If I'd known what was going on at a hormonal level in my brain, it would have helped me to recognise that and make a more conscious effort to relax. And leave the police out of it.

We all have different levels of oxytocin. Just as we're all different for countless reasons. The explanations are unclear. Is it personality? Is it inherited? Is it social support? Or is it a combination of everything and more? We don't know. What we do know is that it is within our control to give it a boost.

The problem with oxytocin is that it's shy. It's the Cinderella of the hormone world. It needs encouragement and it really doesn't have much time for its ugly sisters, adrenaline and cortisol. Both important hormones but at the right time.

When we feel acutely stressed, cortisol and adrenaline spike and put up the hormonal blockers, preventing our oxytocin flow. This is a humdinger of an issue for both feeding and feeling bonded with our babies, which is why the interplay between how we are feeling and our capacity for breastfeeding and connecting with our babies is huge. When we consciously focus on how to create a greater sense of calm, the opposite happens, meaning oxytocin is able to break through and lower the activity in our stress system.

Can't we just pop some oxytocin pills!? Sadly not, at least not at the time of writing. There is an oxytocin spray but to-date there is little research on it and the consensus is that its strength is somewhat reduced anyhow by the time it travels in through the nose and hits the brain cells.

Nevertheless, there are ample simple routes for everyone in the family to take, most of which are relevant regardless of whether you are breastfeeding or formula-feeding, to help ooze the oxytocin.

The beauty of breathing

Why would we need to think about something that we've done automatically billions of times from the moment we were born!? Because breathing is the true link between keeping our bodies and minds on tip-top form and *how* we breathe is fundamental to it all, as Nikki tells us here.

Nikki's Zen Zone

Breathe through it

When we're worried, nervous or anxious, the fear centre in our brain (the amygdala) triggers a whole series of physical responses in our body. Our breathing gets shorter, our heart rate increases and often we sweat. We also tend to be more reactive, feel jittery and struggle to relax.

When we're feeling like this, instructions such as 'just breathe' don't feel very empowering. But taking your breathing into your control is one of the quickest ways to take the edge off things. Why? Because when we regulate our breath, we tap into our body's natural relaxation system, also known as the 'parasympathetic nervous system'.

So here's a handy Zen tool. I'd like you to take three deep purposeful breaths, focusing on breathing out for longer than you breathe in. You can count if you like – in for 4, out for 8. If this works for you, you can continue for a bit longer and try using the out-breath as a tool for breathing a little more space into your tense spots like the jaw and the shoulders.

Go to: www.100fzen.com/awareness and listen to 'Breathe and Come Back'.

Strip off

Many researchers who have devoted years to researching oxytocin, believe the power of skin-to-skin contact with your baby is *the* most significant thing that parents can do to increase both their levels of oxytocin and those of their baby. In practice, snuggling your naked baby (albeit with a nappy to avoid disaster!) on your bare chest, is often encouraged immediately after birth, but very little is spoken about the benefits of doing it at any point further on down the line. Much less, it is scarcely *ever* mentioned to parents who are bottle-feeding.

It's such a simple act and yet whole books have been written about it. The close connection with the baby triggers the release of oxytocin in not only the parent but also the baby. As well as the calming effects this can have, it also helps a baby stabilise their temperature, breathing rate, heart rate and blood-sugar level. When you're at home, a manageable way of having hands-free skin-to-skin time, so that you can still get up, have a pee and move about, is by using a wrap or carrier. So, snuggle away people.

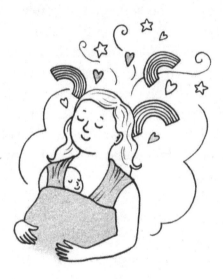

The Hypno*boobing* Effect

The practice of hypno*birthing* is based on the notion that when a woman feels confident, positive and calm during her labour and birth, using:

- the breath
- mindfulness meditation
- positive affirmations
- visualisations

her body has a far greater capacity to be flooded with oxytocin. This hormone in turn leads to the uterus contracting more effectively and allows the woman to experience less distress, exhaustion and pain. Using these same techniques, adapted to be relevant to breast-feeding and the postnatal period (explored throughout this book), can help to boost milk supply, milk flow and a mother's overall sat-isfaction with their breastfeeding experience. I like to call this the hypno*boobing* effect and use this with my clients with great results.

Focusing on a mental activity, such as concentrating hard on a work task whilst breastfeeding, has been shown to decrease oxy-tocin and thereby put the brakes on milk flow, especially in the early days and weeks. Allowing our minds to let go and surrender into the moment is the golden antidote to this and you will notice the instant calm it can bring. It's neither self-indulgent, embar-rassing or a waste of time. It's self-preservation, self-protection and will not only serve to benefit you but everyone around you as well, including predominantly your baby. You will find one of my short hypnoboobing meditation scripts for helping to settle into a calm feeding session on page 142.

Invest in Rest

Resting doesn't necessarily mean sleep. It's really an approach to everyday life. When we feel more rested, our stress response quiet-ens down, the oxytocin flows and sleep itself, when it's available, comes more easily.

Long gone are the 10-day hospital stays after the birth, with matron bustling about, keeping visitors at bay and ushering mothers back into bed. Following an uncomplicated hospital birth these days, you are likely to be home within 24 hours and often far less. It's then easy to get caught up in the adrenaline of the moment and strangely find yourself making tea for visitors before you've barely even man-aged to wash or won the much-maligned battle-of-the-first-poo.

It's often only with hindsight that parents who've been through it before look back and think, What were we thinking having people over for lunch/going to a party/having an open house for a free-for-all gawp!? I put myself firmly in this category as someone who wound up at a wedding (4 hours from home), a mere 2 weeks after giving birth to our first baby and spent the night on a sofa-bed with 6 alcohol-fuelled friends. Ummmm . . . *hello*!? Everything ached. I cried a lot. It was a rubbish idea.

Baby burnout, or simply running out of steam after a few weeks or months, is a bona fide issue and yet is totally avoidable.

Motherhood is the rest of your life, so allowing a few weeks to hole up and have no expectations beyond recovery and adapting to your new set up is more than OK. The world can and will wait.

Steph

The newborn period is the time to go slow. The time to transport your new little family away into a baby bubble as much as you feel and *for as long* as you feel you want and are able to. I'm never going to say 'sleep when the baby sleeps' because, quite frankly, it's irritating to so many people and I can understand why. Your baby has just fallen asleep. Quite likely on you. It's highly possible no one else is around to hold them, so there you are stuck on the sofa, held hostage by your tiny (and cute) captor.

Be pragmatic in times like these. Bring in the reserves as much as you can, especially on any trickier days. Often these days are the ones we hide away, harbouring skewed views of how we *should* be coping on our own. These are the days that should be about shouting 'I need you!' from the rooftops. Ask them to bring over a meal, put on a wash or simply be there for a hug. If family aren't an option and you're able to afford it, investing in some form of paid help in the early weeks, such as a postnatal doula, could help make you feel like a whole different person.

I wished I had slowed down. I'd replaced busy work with busy mothering and had a full timetable of baby yoga, swim, cinema . . . I loved it but I wish I had just had lazy days of dozing and cuddling too.

Lucy

Nikki's Zen Zone

Go kindly on your tired brain
When our brain cells haven't had the renewal from sleep they need, both our mental abilities and our mood are affected. When we're functioning in a haze of insufficient sleeping, it's normal not to be at our best and for anxious thoughts to creep in.

This is a gentle reminder to go kindly on yourself on your more tired days. We usually do our very best to fight our tiredness because, let's face it, it's not a feeling anyone enjoys. Perhaps try instead softening into your tiredness a little and asking yourself this question, 'What one thing could I do to look after myself right now?'

If you're a visual person, you could also try this. Sit down for a moment and imagine you have a heavy weight in each hand. One of them represents productivity and the other one represents perfection. Imagine slowly putting each of these weights down by your sides. And then spend a moment sensing the connection you're making with the bed, chair or sofa and say, 'I hold myself in this moment.'

Go to: www.100fzen.com/emotions and listen to 'Coping With Tiredness'.

If you feel excessively tired there may well be a reason for it beyond 'I've just had a baby' and this warrants looking into. Being anaemic or having a thyroid imbalance (an issue which is renowned for being under-diagnosed postnatally) can have a negative influence on milk supply if you're breastfeeding, as well as adding to feeling like a zombie, so be sure to get tested if you're concerned.

Having postnatal depression or coping with trauma is also known to impact significantly on sleep and energy levels – and this goes for fathers and partners just as much as mothers. It's often assumed that the baby is causing this exhaustion, whereas the key underlying reason could be in how you are feeling. Depression and trauma can affect the time it takes to get to sleep and also how much time you spend awake and being restless during the night.

Embrace the nights

There's no sugar-coating it. Night waking is simply a fact of life with a baby around and no, you are never by any stretch 'failing' at the job if your 1-month-old, 4-month-old or 2-year-old is waking up. Endless worrying about sleep (or the lack of) can be far more exhausting than the acknowledgement that it is normal and not something to battle against. That said, there is plenty you can do to help encourage sleep where you feel you need to (see pages 130–33 for more on this).

As for general ways in helping you get through these nights, you can try the following:

- The least disruptive and safest way to breastfeed in the night is to bring your baby into bed* and learn to feed in a side-lying position. This avoids having to sit up or get out of bed and means that you can rest easy knowing that if you close your eyes and have a snooze, your baby is in a safe position on the mattress. The worry with sitting up in the night is that if a mother drifts off to sleep, the baby could slip down with their face becoming dangerously positioned against her body and/ or cushions.
- If you prefer, or need, to sit up in bed or on a chair for night-time feeds or expressing sessions, keep busy by listening to a podcast, messaging your fellow nocturnal friends with babies or anything else that resonates with

---

* Be sure to read up about safer bed-sharing in Chapter 4.

you, so that you feel reassured that you won't fall asleep
and are not quite so alone at the same time.

- If you're bottle-feeding, be organised in the evenings
  with all the things you need in your bedroom, to avoid
  tiring trips to the kitchen.
- Have a stash of snacks and a water bottle next to you,
  ready for the midnight munchies.
- Keep a changing mat and a few nappies in your bedroom
  so that any changes can be done quickly on your bed
  rather than having to move to a separate room.
- Try to avoid turning on lights. Have a nightlight for your
  room and/or the light on in the hallway outside. If you
  need more light to see what's going on more clearly, keep
  it on for the shortest time possible.
- See Nikki's Zen Zone on page 137 for staying positive
  during long nights.

Be perfectly imperfect

That's not a typo. Striving to reach a mythical level of 'perfect'
parenting is stressful, exhausting and fruitless because it's meaningless and therefore unattainable. What it does set us up for is
the dreaded guilt and sense of failure we feel when we see our path
being different to someone else's. As psychotherapist Anna Mathur
so eloquently writes:

> Guilt does to your mind what pain does to your body. It eats you
> up, steals your peace. It's a price to pay, especially when guilt
> isn't even justified.

So hold your head high, listen to your instinct and notice
when the uncalled-for comparison between yourself and others
creeps in. You are keeping another human alive and that is huge,
regardless of what baby classes you're making it to or how feeding is going.

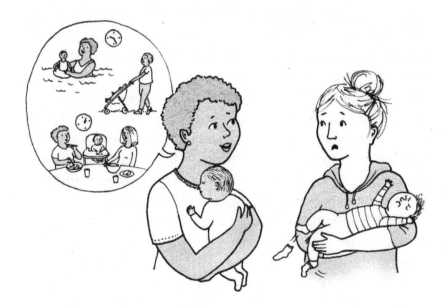

As and when the doubt creeps in, gently remind yourself that it's OK not to always know the answers. You are human. None of us are on telepathic speed dial to The. Ultimate. Answer. Notice what this little pause brings up for you. Are you especially hungry? Tired? Thinking of all your to-dos? Fed up? All the above!? Use this insight to propel yourself onwards into a small action that will reduce this load for you. Perhaps it's a quick snack, a cat nap, answering an email or simply watching the clouds change shape and move in the sky. Whatever it is, giving yourself these mini gifts of brain space will help you to figure out what feels right or wrong for you in any given situation.

Remind yourself that you care so much because you are already a loving and brilliant parent, recognise each little accomplishment you make and fly the flag for being perfectly imperfect.

Pounce on pain

Living with pain after you've had a baby is exceptionally hard and notably takes a toll on emotional resilience and stress levels.

Pain can manifest itself for a whole heap of reasons, from acute (short-term) pain from stitches, after-pains* or figuring out breast-feeding, to less common chronic (longer-term) pain in the back, migraines or pelvic area. Taking over-the-counter medications such as paracetamol and ibuprofen are safe regardless of how you are feeding your baby. If you are prescribed any opiod medication (such as tramadol, co-codamol or codeine), this is still compatible with breastfeeding but should be closely monitored and limited to the shortest reasonable time expected for managing your symptoms (for your health equally as much as the baby's).

Not initiating breastfeeding after birth, or needing to stop abruptly at any point, can lead to painful, swollen breasts for some women. Use plenty of ice packs to help reduce any swelling and take anti-inflammatory pain relief such as ibuprofen. You can find more on ending breastfeeding on page 202.

Finding grace in your body and getting back on the move

When we step back and think about what our body does to bring a baby into our arms, it's hard not to be in awe of its strength, beauty and power. Every new stretch mark, wrinkly bit of skin, tired-looking belly button and dose of cellulite that might come our way, deserves to be honoured because they hold such a very precious story. So if the mini-mind-beasts come knocking to say something contrary, remind yourself that you can always be in control of them and with a good dose of positive self-talk you can send them packing.

Once you feel ready, even gentle exercise is well-established for its benefits on our mood and lowering stress. Taking a short walk outdoors may be the only planned activity you do in a day but will almost guarantee to lift your spirits and help to calm your mind.

---

* After-pains refer to the sensation of the uterus contracting back down into the pelvis in the early days after birth. This is often felt most intensely during breast-feeding, as it's the oxytocin at work again. This feeling can be very mild or extremely painful, like nasty period pains.

When I asked 90 new mothers what they did, or wished they'd done more of in the early months, a staggering 74 per cent of them wrote the simple act of taking a walk.

How do we know when it's safe and what's appropriate to start anything more strenuous? Nicki Philips, founder of the Niix fitness app, gives us her view:

Whether you are keen to get back to exercise or not, it's important to be mindful of the physiological and anatomical changes your body has been through during pregnancy and childbirth. Hormones, muscles, ligaments, bones and your circulatory system have all been affected and need time to readjust.

Before taking up any exercise, I would always recommend that you are signed off by your doctor first and, secondly, if you are able to, have a women's health specialist (such as a physiotherapist or qualified pre- and postnatal Pilates teacher) assess you for any muscle separation, pelvic weakness or pain and postural alignment concerns. All of these are often overlooked, meaning they can go undiagnosed and leave mothers needlessly in discomfort or without strength and stability for a long time.

Social media and our own pressures to get back in shape, often paper over these incredible changes our bodies have been through. It assumes we should snap back into shape, get straight back into pounding the treadmill or pedalling like a champ in a spin class.

Re-educating muscle memory and focusing on key areas such as the pelvic floor, glutes and deep core muscles will ensure a safe return to fitness by building strong foundations. High impact sessions should be avoided until those building blocks have been mastered.

For breastfeeding mamas, moderate exercise does not affect how much milk you have or what's in your milk. However, hard-core training most likely will take its toll over time, so keep your eye out for signs that perhaps your supply is being affected and step back a little if you can and want to. To keep yourself comfortable whilst exercising, aim to feed beforehand, so that you're not feeling quite so full. If your little one wants a feed as soon as you're done, they may prefer it if you give your breast a quick rinse to wash away any salty, sweaty taste.

Eat and drink happy

It's a well-known fact that what we eat and drink is central to how we feel physically and emotionally. Though living with a new baby doesn't exactly lend itself to giving you much time (if any!) to consider this. Laura Clark, a registered dietician, shares her top tips:

> It can be tempting to cut calories to lose some baby weight but this can quickly zap a new mother of energy and negatively affect her milk supply. What will make the most difference is eating well to avoid cravings for high sugar and high fat foods.
>
> Try to keep to a regular meal pattern and combine protein and carbs together to help regulate your blood-sugar levels and reduce your reliance on stimulants like caffeine. If main meals are difficult, snacks can be just as wholesome, for example oatcakes and peanut butter, wholemeal pitta with hummus, popcorn and cheese, nuts and dried fruit, malt loaf or pulses like flavoured peas. All these snacks have fibre in them too which will help keep your bowels healthy and moving.
>
> Consider making dinners with brown rice, bulgur wheat or wholemeal couscous. The grains bind together when served with some veggies and oily fish like salmon, topped off with some natural yoghurt and herbs – perfect to eat with one hand! The same goes for risotto or cottage pie with plenty of pulses in it.
>
> Combining slow release carbs with some protein and fibre will encourage tryptophan to enter your brain, which works to

help you sleep. When you can sleep, make it count by having a sleepy snack beforehand. A bowl of wholegrain cereal with milk or peanut butter on toast is the perfect combination to boost magnesium levels, which also help muscles to relax.

Remember to hydrate, hydrate, hydrate! Being dehydrated is hell for keeping a straight mind and energised body. Starting the day with a glass of water on waking is a sure-fire way to kick the day off positively and help avoid feeling like an abandoned pot plant by mid-morning.

Just being

Having time just 'to be', with or without the baby, is fundamental to reducing the overwhelm that can hit us all. It may be that you feel 'touched out' and just can't deal with any more physical contact at that moment. Or the monotony of your day with a young baby starts to feel lonely and overbearing.

Notice whether a scroll on social media gives you a boost or makes you feel wobbly and try to adjust your habits and people you follow accordingly. During a feed have a think about ringing a good friend, watching a boxset (even better if it's a laugh-out-loud one), meditating, reading a magazine or book, or listening to a favourite podcast or album. Whilst things you can do either with (easier in a sling) or without your baby could be gentle yoga, walking, playing an instrument, lighting some candles and having a relaxing bath, working, singing or meeting friends for a drink.

I didn't allow my babies out of my sight and I learnt by number three that it was OK to leave someone else watching the baby, so I could nap or do something for myself for a short while and they could get me if the baby woke up. But that did take me three babies to work out!

Alice

Ponder point

Whatever it may be, take a moment to write down and reflect on what it is that's important to you just 'to be' and list what is achievable.

Now:

In the next few weeks:

In the next few months:

Just by writing it down and realising that some things, no matter how small, *are* manageable, can help boost a mood even before doing any of it!

I went out a lot and met up with NCT friends. They were a great tonic and a lot of fun. I also joined several baby classes. People would say that they found maternity leave tough because of the lack of adult conversation and the lack of intellectual stimulation. I found it far from lacking in either. I've never had so much time to socialise (once we were over the early days) and conversation with the other mums would range from nappies to politics, history, culture and back to nappies again!

Jen

Go gently on relationships

If you are in a relationship, you may not be surprised to learn that having a young family is frequently cited as being right up there as one of the top causes of stress between couples. We're tired, busy and emotions run high for all sorts of reasons.*

If my friends and I are anything to go by it's OK and perfectly normal to intermittently want to shoot your partner for anything/everything/nothing/breathing. It will pass and you most likely did choose the right person but the transition into parenthood is very different for mothers and fathers, and tiredness and hormones are responsible for a lot!

Tilly

Consequently, it's not uncommon for healthy communication to start slipping down the drain. These women have some sage words:

---

* If any relationship struggles you are having run deeper than this, and particularly if you ever feel threatened, controlled or have been hurt in any way, know that you are *never* to blame, regardless of what you may have been told and may currently believe. Telling someone you trust about what is going on, such as a friend, your GP or health visitor, only represents how strong you are and is the first step to a life that you deserve.

Don't panic if you feel like your relationship has turned upside down. I remember going to a breastfeeding clinic with a friend when our partners were on paternity leave. Her husband wrapped his arm around her as she fed, while mine nodded off in the chair. I felt so scared and disconnected that having a baby wasn't this uniting experience that it so obviously was with my friends, but all we needed was time to get through the absolute chaos that was looking after a newborn. Give yourself time to adjust but try and have some form of physical contact every day, even if it's just a quick cuddle or a shoulder squeeze.

Chelsea

Have fun with each other, laugh about little mishaps and let your partner do things their way. I tried to be too controlling but once I changed my mindset, I was able to enjoy my husband and my baby more.

Lauren

Nikki's Zen Zone

I forgive you and I forgive me

Whether it's a misjudged comment or a tiger-style roar, when we're tired and under pressure we snap. We can be more quick to feel hurt by others and to hurt others too. We all move on from these hurtful moments in different ways but if we don't acknowledge and let go of the difficulty, it usually lingers or snowballs into something else.

Many of us set the bar so high for ourselves and others that making mistakes doesn't sit comfortably. However, simply realising that we're fallible beings, all capable of doing hurtful things we regret, can help to keep things in perspective.

Forgiveness is an act of kindness towards yourself, a sign of strength rather than weakness. Imagine how tenderly you would talk to a young child who had made a mistake and see if you can offer some gentleness towards the hurt you're feeling. Allow yourself to feel it and be with it and try offering these words quietly to yourself, 'I forgive you and I forgive me'.

And what of sex? Only you know when the time is right again, depending on both your physical recovery, general mental wellness and energy. I asked clinical psychologist Karen Gurney (aka The Sex Doctor) what her top tips are:

My number one tip is don't be mistaken that if your sex life takes a turn for the worse that it means there is something wrong with you or your relationship. Some sex therapists call this period of having small children the 'do no harm' years with regards to your sex life. This basically refers to the fact that although things may dip, it's important to retain as much physical and emotional intimacy as you can during this time, so that a change in your sex life doesn't affect your relationship satisfaction. Making time to share a brief passionate kiss, being naked together without an end goal, ensuring you still compliment each other and making time to connect as a couple (if only very briefly) are key.

It's not inevitable that your sex life will be negatively impacted in this period, it's just common. You may be one of the couples whose sex life gets better, so don't expect the worst! Many couples I have worked with have found their emotional connection, sex life and how they manage their sex life (like making time for it) has been positively impacted upon by having kids, so it's not all doom and gloom!

Breastfeeding can reduce sex drive in some women* and lead to some vaginal dryness (not for all), so, if the moment takes you,

---

* Higher levels of the hormone prolactin keep the level of oestrogen low, which can sometimes result in a reduced sex drive.

have a suitable lubricant handy. These mothers had some other thoughts to add about sex and breastfeeding:

I always wore a bra. Nothing less attractive than having breast milk squirting all over your partner in the middle!

I wasn't bothered about sex for a long time and sleep was way higher on both our agendas. We're slowly getting there now though, fifteen months on.

I made sure I'd fed or expressed just beforehand and had something nearby to catch any escaping milk.

The professionals looking out for you

Even in the UK where we have a standardised pathway of care for postnatal women and babies, it comes down to where you live, who you get and what your circumstances are.

If you are back home within a few days of birth, or had your baby at home, you are likely to see a midwife on day 5 and again around about day 10. If there are any concerns about how things are going, you may be offered additional visits, or be asked to come to a drop-in clinic. Many midwifery teams have midwifery support workers (MSWs) who may be called in to support you with feeding.

Most families will be transferred from the midwifery to the health visiting service around 10–14 days post-birth, who will then be a source of support to you all the way up until your child goes to school. A health visitor is a nurse who has had additional training in child health and development, and family mental and social wellbeing. The point of a health visitor is to support you to be the best parent you can be, so that you and your children are as happy and healthy as possible. They are *not* there to inspect you and snoop around your home or hoping to find you all dressed up, hair done and lipstick on. In fact, if everything does seem too La La Land perfect then they might even worry more.

Use them as often as you wish. Ask them any questions and offload as much as you want. They expect and welcome it. Fathers and partners should always be made to feel welcome at any visit or in any baby clinic. As in any profession, there are many good eggs and others that are off. If at any point, you don't feel comfortable with anything that is said to you, don't ever feel that you must take it as golden. Do your research, chat to friends and seek out other opinions.

You will also have a postnatal check-up with the GP around 6–8 weeks after the birth, who should ask you how things are going, how you are feeling and refer you on to any other services if needs be.

How to know if a health professional is not supportive of what *you* want

Professionals who have been thoroughly trained in infant feeding and counselling skills (and have taken it on board!), will never make anyone feel judged or guilty for breastfeeding, formula-feeding, expressing, mixed-feeding, tube-feeding, cup-feeding or using anything-that-safely-works-feeding.

However, there are a lot of well-meaning people who deem themselves in an appropriate position to offer a supposedly 'educated' opinion, who are sadly misinformed and who tend to be the ones who end up making some women feel pants.

Inconsistent advice and finding it hard to access relevant experts was a huge trigger for me ... I realised I just had to zone out certain people for a while until I felt more confident.

Jonas

The irony of the debate about 'pressure' to breastfeed is that whilst many professionals appear supportive of breastfeeding when it is going well, countless mothers are advised and influenced by these same professionals to either unnecessarily stop breast-feeding or start to add in formula, if and when things start to look tricky. Of course, sometimes this is absolutely necessary and it may well be exactly what the mother wants to do.

The problem however is this: many women stop breastfeeding or introduce some formula when they themselves really *didn't want and need to* and simply because they got bad advice.

So how can you tell if someone is flying the flag for helping you to meet your goals?

- They will not tell you that 'breast is best' and that you just need to 'keep going' if you are clearly struggling and simply 'keeping going' is not cutting the mustard.
- They will get to the root of any problem, explain it fully and plan with you for how to turn things around.
- They will be realistic, sensitive and honest. If things are truly not going to happen in the way you'd originally hoped, despite having taken every step to get there, they will work with you to modify your goals and make a new plan that you feel happy and confident with.
- They will signpost or refer you to more specialist support if the situation is beyond their level of knowledge or training and not make you feel that the buck stops with them and there are no more answers.
- If you have chosen not to breastfeed and feel happy with your decision, they will not try to talk you down. They should help you stay comfortable to avoid developing breast pain or infection and will chat with you about all the ways that you can still maximise bonding with your baby.

Mental health conditions and new parenthood

We've seen that 'new parent anxiety' is common. However, what if more is going on? Some parents, with or without a relevant medical history, can develop generalised anxiety disorder (GAD) or obsessive compulsive disorder (OCD) during pregnancy or in the postnatal period, where anxious and intrusive thoughts become all-encompassing and interfere with everyday life. Additionally, it's not uncommon to be affected by pre- or postnatal depression (PND) or some degree of post-traumatic stress disorder (PTSD), which we will specifically cover here.

Pre- and postnatal depression

PND is a condition whereby the baby blues don't seem to shift after those early weeks and the symptoms start to feel more intense and severe. Studies suggest that around 10–15 per cent of mothers and 10 per cent of fathers in the UK will develop some degree of post-natal depression. Additionally, post-surrogacy and post-adoption depression are also recognised concerns in both men and women, with symptoms mirroring those of PND (although they have some unique causal factors unrelated to pregnancy and birth). If this is affecting you or your partner, you may notice some or all of these additional signs:

- You (or a partner) seem to be 'checking out' from each other and/or other family and close friends
- There are difficulties with feeling bonded to your baby and the day seems to drift by on autopilot
- Feeling tired all the time
- Appetite changes
- Persisting feelings of sadness
- Loss of interest, joy or pleasure in doing things you or a partner would normally enjoy
- There are strong feelings of guilt, shame and/or worthlessness
- It becomes harder and harder to fall asleep
- There may be a preoccupation with thoughts of leaving the family or even with dying

There isn't one simple explanation as to why some people develop PND above others. The reasons are multi-factorial and it is important to know that just because any of these reasons may relate to you, it does not mean that developing PND is inevitable. This is not an exhaustive list but some evidenced-based explanations include:

- Certain life events, such as bereavement, illness (affecting yourself, your baby or anyone else close to you), fertility difficulties, having your baby prematurely, relationship breakdowns or difficulties, historical or current experience of abuse, financial troubles, having little or no family support or moving to an unfamiliar place.
- Having a history of one or more mood disorders such as depression, anxiety, OCD or trauma.
- Hormonal imbalances (potentially exacerbated by pregnancy and birth but may also be related to thyroid or pituitary conditions).
- For some men, other possible factors include feeling a burden of financial responsibility, feeling isolated and lonely, missing their sexual relationship and/or feeling overwhelmed or trapped. Sometimes there may be no clear reason at all.
- Further exacerbating factors are known to be complications in pregnancy, birth or breastfeeding, stopping breastfeeding abruptly, the baby's temperament, high parental expectations of themselves, the change of pace (i.e. being alone at home versus a structured and busy day at work), returning early to work, chronic pain and lack of sleep.

PND blinds you to the obvious. I 'wanted it all' and believe that I ultimately got sick because of it. For me, breastfeeding helped with connecting with my daughter and having time to sit and relax, and stop the anxious fussing. Several times I considered stopping as I thought I may get more rest and recover sooner if I wasn't breastfeeding but I'm so glad we continued.

Jennifer

Very rarely (in approximately 1–2 in 1,000 of all births) women develop a condition known as 'post-natal psychosis'. This is different to PND in that a woman will experience frightening delusional thoughts, confusion and disorientation, and rapid mood swings from huge highs to deep lows. This is recognised as a medical emergency and mothers should be treated rapidly, often with in-patient care and with their baby staying alongside them.

Post-traumatic stress disorder

Trauma is often associated with war veterans or victims of humanitarian or natural disasters. What is less talked about is that trauma symptoms can be caused by *anything* where there is perceived to be an actual or threatened risk of death, injury or violation. The experience of birth and/or postnatal illness can very much come under any of those categories for some parents. Many studies over the last 20 years have found that up to one third of women described their birth as traumatic, and although not all these women will develop ongoing symptoms of trauma, some women (and/or their partners) may go on to recognise the following in themselves:

- Grieving for a birth experience that didn't happen
- Feeling intense fear, horror and helplessness
- Isolating oneself
- Feeling numb and/or hopeless
- Difficulty concentrating and sleeping
- Feeling angry and irritable
- Appearing to overreact to certain situations
- Having flashbacks, nightmares and even hallucinations

Research of women's experiences tells us that the possible physical and emotional impacts of a traumatic birth can result in a range of very different feelings towards infant feeding. Some women find that if breastfeeding is painful or they are worried about their milk supply, for instance, the ensuing worry can feel like a deeply insurmountable ordeal that could also significantly impact on their ability to feel bonded with their baby. On the other hand, other women discover that a traumatic birth strengthens their desire and determination to breastfeed and find that it can greatly heal their mental hurt and encourage strong attachment to their baby.

This is a very clear example of just how unique we all are and that a blanket one-size-fits-all approach to support for women and their families is only ever going to suit some parents, and will feel alienating and more destructive to others.

What to do if you are worried about yourself or someone close to you

If you are concerned at any point about either your mental health, or that of a partner or anyone else significant to you, the first step towards feeling better is always acknowledging what's going on. Whether that's starting by writing down your feelings, having a gentle and open conversation with a loved one, posting in a private support group on social media, or speaking to your doctor or other health professional, making that first move is a powerful and significant positive step.

Always know that you are NEVER to blame, and feeling this way does not reflect your ability as a mother or father. It *is* possible to make a full recovery from these conditions. They are never something you have to just get on and live with.

If, at any point, you find yourself thinking, I don't want to make a fuss or I'll be wasting their time, take a moment to put a gigantic hypothetical dart through the middle of those thoughts and let them go. No worry is ever too small to chat about.

It felt too self-indulgent to give it too much attention or thought. Nobody spoke to me about my traumatic first birth, even though it was the reason I gave to have an elective c-section for my subsequent delivery. With hindsight I needed help desperately.

Lisa

Depending on your individual circumstances, the road ahead may involve anything from making simple lifestyle changes at home to referrals for professional talking therapies, complementary therapies, medical tests to check for any nutritional deficiencies or hormonal imbalances, possible medication and occasionally in-patient care, such as at a residential mother and baby unit.

It didn't help to be told 'just relax' or 'you're being silly'. What personally helped my anxiety was having things in place like a video monitor . . . However, CBT ultimately taught me ways to self-soothe without seeking reassurance from my partner or anything else.

Ivy

If you are breastfeeding and want to continue, none of these interventions should stand in your way. It is perfectly possible to be on medications that are compatible with breastfeeding (as covered on pages 24), if that is the right course of action for you.

AFFIRMATIONS

- *I listen to my body and my heart and give it what it needs*
- *It is right for me to be kind to myself*
- *I am the best I can be right now and that is good enough*
- *If I feel guilty it doesn't mean that I am guilty*
- *Not loving every moment of parenthood doesn't mean I don't love being a parent*

3

Being a baby – what's going on in their heads?

Knowing how babies think and what they are capable (and not capable) of doing, is fundamental to building an understanding of how and why they feed the way they do. In this chapter we'll look at:

- What's inside a baby's brain
- What a newborn can do to help themselves to feed
- Factors that can affect their ability to feed
- Where we can start with helping babies to feed

Inside a baby's brain

The enormous relative size of our human brains to our bodies sets us apart from every other mammal. Given ideal conditions in which to thrive, our astonishing brains allow us to solve complex problems, to form meaningful relationships, to control our emotions and to live independent lives. But therein lies the problem. If we waited until our brain was sufficiently developed before birth to figure this stuff out, even just a little bit, pregnancy would last for a heck of a lot longer than 9 months. Ouch. Given the narrow size of our hips through which we'd have to birth these babies, plus the metabolic energy it takes to stay pregnant, humanity would have long since given up the ghost.

The result is that our babies are born a long way off from being mini-adults with a conscious stream of thought and a solid understanding about what they need, why they need it and how to go about getting it.

There are crudely three main parts of the brain.

1. The reptilian brain: The automatic control centre at the base of the brain where blood pressure, temperature control, reflexes, breathing rate and heart rate are all set up without any conscious work. In a healthy, term baby this part of the brain is fully functioning, albeit immaturely (which is why a baby has a faster heart beat, for example).

2. The mammalian brain: The mid-brain is where we feel emotion and instinctual drive for things such as hunger, pain, comfort, love and security. As above, this part of the brain is functioning well in a healthy, term baby.

3. The human brain: The frontal cortex or 'higher' brain is where we develop conscious thought and the ability to problem-solve, rationalise, develop language and calm ourselves down, amongst many other skills.

At birth, babies have all the nerve cells present and correct in their human brain that they are ever going to need. The issue is that they aren't connected to anything. Think of billions of homes, built in total isolation from each other, without any roads or pathways linking them and enabling travel. In other words, these cells are floating freely about, not talking to each other, and thus all these complex skills are entirely beyond the capacity of any baby to take on, regardless of whatever potential genius they may grow into.

During the first 2 years of life, their experience of the world and the way in which they are cared for creates billions of synapses (or mini motorways) between these cells to enable the brain to fully fire up and start figuring all this out. Whilst this gradual sophistication of the human brain is happening, babies function predominantly in their reptilian and mammalian brains and thus are driven by automatic and instinctual reactions, as we will now go on to see.

Reflexes and behavioural states

Healthy babies are born primed to search out their source of milk and feed. Amongst others, they have various automatic reflexes that specifically help them to feed if given the chance.

- **Rooting.** When the corner of a baby's mouth is touched, she will turn her head and open her mouth to 'root' in the direction of the touch. This helps her to search out the source of her 'food', which can also manifest in her bobbing her head about (it's incredible how strong their neck muscles are in order to help with this searching behaviour). When the rooting reflex is stimulated this often causes babies to suck on their hands or fingers.
- **Stepping.** This is often referred to as the walking or dancing reflex as it looks like a baby is taking steps when held upright and their feet touch a solid surface. When held in certain positions on a mother's body, this reflex also enables her to search out the breast and start to feed.
- **Grasping.** When she feels something against her hands she will grasp it. This helps her to familiarise herself with where she is. Her favourite thing to grasp? You!
- **Sucking.** When the roof of her mouth is gently stimulated by touch, she will begin to suck, whether this be on a breast, bottle teat, finger or dummy.

Together with these reflexes, newborn babies also display identifiable behavioural states that will either help put them in the mood to feed or not.

- **Quiet sleep** (deep sleep). She is completely conked out. She may stir very slightly but remains pretty much unresponsive to noise or movement.
- **Active sleep** (light sleep). She may startle to sudden noises, twitch her limbs, move her mouth and her eyes may move rapidly underneath closed eyelids (even occasionally opening and closing quickly).
- **Drowsiness.** The stage between waking up or falling asleep. She may have droopy eyelids, yawn, stretch and generally look a little dazed.
- **Quiet alert.** She makes small and infrequent movements, lying quite still with open eyes. She may make eye contact, turn to noises and copy facial expressions.
- **Active alert.** She fusses a little, kicks her arms and legs and starts to be vocal (e.g. making cooing noises).
- **Crying.** She may fuss loudly now. This is often through increased hunger, tiredness, frustration, discomfort or loneliness.

Babies will be able to feed calmly and most effectively when they are either in states of active sleep, drowsiness or quiet alertness. Trying to feed a baby when they are either in quiet sleep or a crying state is certainly trickier.

Reflexes and behavioural states are not a readily given constant for every single baby; your baby may vary depending on the following.

Being born early

Reflexes start to develop between 28–32 weeks of pregnancy and do not fully develop until around 36 weeks. Therefore, babies born early will usually have a weak or immature sucking pattern and need some extra help to feed. Preterm babies also spend more time asleep and will often feed more slowly, need waking a little for feeds and feed little and often. As they will have had less time to build up body fat, regular skin contact whenever possible with their caregiver will help them to control their temperature, keeping them snuggly warm and primed for feeding.

Born with additional neurological and/or medical needs

Babies born with a condition or disorder that may affect their physical or neurological ability to feed without additional support, may include those with respiratory or heart problems, cerebral palsy, gastro-intestinal disorders, head and neck abnormalities, cleft lip and/or palate and Down's syndrome (this is not an exhaustive list). With all these conditions, babies will be under the care of specialist teams who will support and advise each family individually.

The process of birth

Whilst some babies are ready to feed within the first hour of birth, others can be sleepy and take a little while to get going and wake up to the world. This is more common if babies have pain-relieving medication, such as pethidine, in their system, that has passed through the umbilical cord and thus causes them to be a little drowsy when they come earth-side. Other mechanical interventions such as forceps and ventouse, or any other source of additional pressure on a baby's skull, whether it be from their positioning in the womb or possible handling of the baby as they are being born, can also instigate a slightly slower start, as Emma Hayward, specialist paediatric osteopath, explains:

> Their position in-utero can affect tension in their body. For example, if a baby engages very early, they can find their head stays stuck in one position for a few weeks. This can sometimes make their necks less able to turn to both sides [a condition called Torticollis]. This can often be picked up when the baby prefers to feed from one breast or one part of their head begins to flatten.
>
> The birth itself can also affect tension in the body. A very

long or very quick birth can put the baby and the mother under more strain. Babies that have had a long birth or experienced an instrumental delivery can be quite 'squashed', less able to move their neck and jaw or find they have a tight side or asymmetry. Both birth and inter-uterine positioning can affect the positioning of the bones of the head.

Osteopathic treatment helps the body function better by improving alignment and reducing areas of tension and discomfort. Cranial techniques are very gentle and help the body to relax and to realign different areas of tension so they feel comfortable and work well.

Human practice

When a kitten or a puppy is born, what do we do? If they are healthy, the answer is, not a huge amount. We leave them be. Snuggled up close to their mother without anything in their way, so they can stay warm, feel safe and feed as and when they want.

This is where, for all our impressive human brain power, we have historically (in Western culture) over-thought and over-complicated what we do with a human baby once they're born. Looking back at parenting books of the early twentieth century it becomes clear that emerging thought about how best to care for a newborn baby only served to screw up rather a lot for babies, who weren't exactly in a position to stand up for themselves and say, 'Hey, what are you doing this for!?' Parents were encouraged to bathe their baby immediately, dress them, wrap them and keep them in a separate cot (or even better, in a separate room). Babies were then brought to their mother at specific 'feeding times' and if they were to be breastfed, a complex process ensued of exposing a tiny bit of breast and having the swaddled baby's head rather roughly pushed towards the target by a kindly yet forthright midwife! It is little wonder that these practices, ignoring what we now know about reflexes and behavioural states, coincided with a significant decline in breastfeeding rates.

What we can do to make the most of reflexes and behavioural states

There are many tricks that we, as parents, can pull out of the bag to help support babies to utilise their reflexes and behavioural states effectively to help feeding progress smoothly.

Skin-to-skin

Here it is again! Babies need to know instinctively that they are in a safe, happy place and not feel under any pressure to get on with it. And this is where skin-to-skin contact comes in again. Touch is often referred to as 'the mother of all senses' because the skin is both our largest sensory organ and the first one to develop in the womb. When this touch is loving and positive, it sends powerful messages to the brain to release oxytocin. As a result, the baby's body will spend less energy on keeping stress and inflammation at bay and have a whole lot more energy spare to spend on building healthy and positive synapses in the brain. With this sensitive touch (and this includes stroking, kissing, massage, carrying and so on), children have the optimal chance for these synapses to build secure and self-confident brains, with greater resilience to dealing with stress. Even though we have no conscious memory of this early time in our lives, these happy experiences become stored in our brains as emotional memory before our brains are mature enough to store them as memories we can recall. These emotional memories underlie our image of the world as a safe place and help to build the type of person we are to become. Effects that truly last a lifetime.

When she is held skin-to-skin with her mother in a slightly reclined position, she is far more able to use her innate reflexes and instinct to start to feed, which paints a stark contrast to a wrapped up baby plonked on a tiny area of exposed nipple!

In the first couple of weeks, spending at least an hour a day or more skin-to-skin means that she:

- Is more likely to latch on well
- Maintains her normal body temperature better even than in an incubator
- Maintains her normal heart rate, respiratory rate and blood pressure
- Has higher blood sugar
- Is less likely to cry
- Is more likely to breastfeed exclusively and breastfeed longer
- Is more likely to clearly indicate to her mother when she is ready to feed

Discover their cues

It would be handy if young babies could talk but of course they don't. Or, at least, not in the way we generally think of talking. When I was a student nurse I was taught that babies communicate by crying. They cry if they're tired, hungry, dirty or whatever. Easy. What I came to realise over the years, however, is that babies are a lot more sophisticated than many give them credit for. Babies have numerous, often subtle, signals that they use to 'talk' and communicate to us what they need and when, way before they lose the plot entirely.

Overleaf are a few common baby cues. You may see some or all of them in your baby.

Common baby cues

	Tired	Hungry	Over-stimulated	Bored and/or lonely	Windy
EARLY CUES	Rubbing eyes	Smacking or sucking sounds, licking lips	Seems cranky/fussy	Fussing which quickly calms with friendly interaction such as cuddles, rocking, singing and eye contact	Quiet gazing and/or 'smiling' (in babies younger than 6 weeks). The smile may be just a flutter and the gaze may indicate the baby is stopping wind that is stopping her falling asleep
	Yawning	Rooting, opening mouth and sticking out tongue	Rubbing eyes		Rooting – a baby may want to feed to help discomfort from wind
	'Checking out', avoiding eye contact or looking dazed and 'glazed'	Sucking on anything – hands, fingers, blankets, Dad's ears! (After 6–8 weeks this is not a reliable sign of hunger; she will explore anything she can with her mouth to learn about the world)	Turning away from you repeatedly and getting agitated by playful interactions. She's trying to say 'not now thanks, I'm done!'		

LATER CUES	Getting fussy: jerky movements of her limbs, moving her head quickly	Fidgeting and squirming around trying to find milk	May either become drowsy (trying to zone out) or become overly attentive to what is happening. The difference here is that her body will be stiff and tense (rather than relaxed in a normal active way)	Increasingly agitated but will again respond well to friendly interaction	Becoming fussy or agitated on the breast or bottle
LAST DITCH CUES	Crying	Crying	Crying	Crying	Crying
	Being awake for longer than her normal acceptable timeframe	Frantic, agitated movements			Arching back. Clenched fists, flexed feet and increasing colour in her face. Possible vomiting

Respond to cues

In relation to feeding, some babies naturally fall into a seemingly textbook pattern of feeding from early on (I would question which 'textbook' this is exactly!) and predictably show feeding cues at regular intervals. However, to burst this bubble, it rarely lasts consistently. It was parenting manuals from the nineteenth century that introduced the idea of strict, scheduled feeds, to fit in with workers' hours, which contributed to a rapid decline in breastfeeding rates.

From an evolutionary viewpoint, we are simply not designed to go for long and equally-spaced intervals between feeds. One look back at the developmental immaturity of a baby's brain and the speed at which it is growing, explains why human milk has evolved to be drunk frequently as a regular energy hit and ensure that the baby is never far from adult protection. Moreover, it takes just a second to reflect on how we eat from toddlerhood through to adulthood, to see that we all eat and drink at fairly random times and consume differing amounts, depending on the day, how we feel, how hot or cold it is and how bored or stimulated we are. Sometimes it's a snacky-can't-really-be-bothered-to-eat-properly kind of a day and other days we may be ravenous and have larger more spaced-out meals, interspersed with a few drinks here and there.

Healthy, term babies intrinsically know what they need and when they need it. In case you hear anything to the contrary, this includes the fact that breast milk has evolved to help babies feel relaxed and sleepy when they need to rest, and thus 'allowing' a baby to breastfeed to sleep is biologically normal, despite what you may otherwise be told. If *you* don't have a problem with it, your baby certainly won't either.

For the babies who can't give us feeding cues, they aren't going to 'demand' to be fed and, as such, can miss out on vital feeding time. Therefore, we want to scrap the term *feeding on demand* (commonly used in the baby world) and replace it with *responsive feeding*. Feeding 'responsively' means responding to both a baby's needs, whether they are making cues for it or not, and to the mother's needs (so if your breasts are about to explode then by all means encourage the baby to feed).

Responsive feeding means that:

- Bottle-fed babies tend to benefit by having less wind and constipation, as a result of having smaller, slightly more frequent feeds.
- Breastfed babies also tend to have few issues with wind and general discomfort as they will be benefiting from lower volume, yet higher fat milk.
- Breastfeeding mothers are more likely to establish a good milk supply (as their brains are getting unrestricted signals to keep making more).
- It also helps all babies, regardless of being on a bottle or breast, to regulate their own appetites, setting them up brilliantly for healthier eating patterns throughout their life.
- Research has also shown that babies fed responsively can have higher IQ scores and experience less stress, and even pain (e.g. during an injection), than strictly schedule-fed babies, making a positive life-long imprint on their rapidly developing brains. Jiggling a crying baby around or leaving them on their own to cry, with the goal of stretching their feeds apart, is very likely to not only be stressful for the baby but also the caregiver. By the time the baby gets to feed, she will likely be tired and frustrated and this generally serves to make feeding time trickier.
- Parents can best meet their baby's needs to feel safe, warm and loved during any periods of illness or otherwise, by providing comfort and nutrients as and when needed (as well as immune-boosting properties if it is breast milk).

My mother was adamant about the 4-hour routine, and my
mother-in-law and stepmother had the same opinion. I would
get comments like, 'She cannot possibly be hungry again' and
insinuations that it was my fault she fed little and often instead
of longer feeds at greater gaps. I had a remarkable ability to rely
on my instincts and shut out this advice. I can't say anything
other than I just 'knew' that what I was doing was the right
thing for us.

Tabitha

Responsive feeding does NOT mean that you will be spoiling your baby, that she will be clingy or that she will never learn how to sleep independently. Let any such inferences you hear simply pass you by.

Falling asleep towards the end of a feed, particularly on the breast, is a physiologically normal response for a baby and does not mean that you are doing anything 'wrong'. *If* you would like to gently encourage her to fall asleep independent of sucking, remember that this can take time and if it isn't happening then she may simply not be ready quite yet.

Parents of twins, triplets and more have different tactics in how they approach responsive feeding and generally make it through the day! Some parents will wait for one baby to wake and soon after wake the second baby so that they can be fed at the same time (whether this is on the breast or bottle). Others prefer to let the first baby have their feed and then gently encourage the second baby to feed close afterwards, if they haven't already woken spontaneously. Other parents will go totally with the flow and feed fully in response to each of their baby's individual cues. See the Resource section at the back of the book for some fabulous places to go for free information and peer support specifically on the practicalities and realities of feeding multiples.

Take time to watch your own baby's unique cues, which will help you to help them. Some days it may be obvious what she's up to and other days you will feel clueless about the flipping cues. It is normal to feel this way so try not to berate yourself. There may well be times too that the *only* cue really does seem to be crying, as she goes from take-off to the moon in a nano-second. Gradually you will see patterns emerging and the predictability of the day becomes easier to judge and manage.

When I felt at a loss about what he needed to calm down I just stuck him on the boob. It worked most of the time. When it didn't I soon realised it was usually due to wind or that he was so over tired that feeding seemed to stimulate him more ... then he'd normally settle once he was in the sling and being walked about.

Ailsa

Ponder point

Writing down what cues you feel you are starting to see in your baby can help you begin to decipher your own baby's 'language'.

AFFIRMATIONS

- *I trust that my baby's cues show instinctive needs and not deliberate control over me*
- *My baby is a beautifully unique soul that I try not to compare with others*

4

Sleep, settling and the link to feeding

The need to address sleep is central in order to get a handle on feeding. I am *not* referring to getting into schedules and sleep training. This is about figuring out what is normal for her, understanding what she needs (and what works for you) and having some tricks up your sleeve to help smooth things along. In this chapter I will provide you with a little insight into:

- Why and how babies sleep the way they do
- Why babies can display common 'fussy' behaviours
- Recognising when there may be additional challenges present such as reflux or allergies
- What we can do as parents to help all babies settle well and thereby feed better

Remember: babies are dynamic. They change hour by hour and day by day. Being open to flexibility could take a huge weight off your shoulders and increase your resilience to stress, particularly on trickier days. Just because you start off doing one thing, doesn't mean you have to stick with it. Parenting is always about discovery and changing things as you go, if it feels right.

The ins and outs of baby sleep

Baby brains are developing at the speed of light and most of this is going on whilst they are asleep. In addition, sleep boosts the immune system, increases growth and ultimately re-sets the baby so that they are happy and calm to feed and experience the world. Gradually establishing sleep patterns that fit for your individual baby undoubtedly has benefits for her and the whole family in reducing irritability, supporting her brain development, developing her circadian rhythm, encouraging better feeding and, importantly, helping everyone to feel that little bit more chilled out.

How babies sleep

How a baby sleeps is markedly different to how we sleep at every other phase in our life. Most notably, babies have much shorter sleep cycles than adults (around 30–40 minutes for a newborn vs 90–120 minutes for adults) and spend considerably more time in lighter sleep. As an adult we are generally unaware of transitioning from one sleep cycle to the next – we roll over, pull up the duvet, twitch, reach for some water or maybe go to the toilet. For a baby, it takes time for this consolidation of sleep to happen and for good reason.

> **Building brains.** Overall, babies spend more time in light sleep because this is when they are processing all their new sensory experiences and speedily making the neural connections in their brains.

> **Survival.** When a baby is in lighter sleep they are less vulnerable to sudden infant death syndrome (SIDS) than if they were to spend longer periods in a deep sleep, requiring greater stimulation to wake up. From an evolutionary perspective, it is thought that these wake-ups were also designed to keep

the mother and baby hormonally in-sync with each other and thus ensure that the baby is protected.

Needing naps. Sleeping during the day not only helps to process memories and consolidate learning but also helps to regulate their heart rate, breathing and body temperature, thus strengthening their immune system. Having a nap also helps to keep babies calmer.

Hunger. Newborn babies have very small stomachs, and need to feed often, so they may wake at least every 2–3 hours in order to do so, and sometimes more often. As babies grow they are able to happily go longer between feeds.

What makes babies go to sleep (and stay awake)

We can tempt ourselves to eat something even when we're not hungry, or push ourselves to go for a run even if we're tired. We can't, however, tell ourselves to suddenly fall asleep if we're not tired. Likewise, feeling stressed or anxious about going to sleep, even if we're exhausted, often makes our brains and bodies fight against it. This is because sleep is not something that we have fully under our conscious control.

Sleep is regulated by two systems:

1. **Sleep-wake homeostasis**

This refers to the system that balances our body's need to sleep, often referred to as sleep pressure. It is regulated by the biochemical rise and fall of substances in the fluid around the brain and spinal cord. The longer we have been awake the more these build up and the need (or pressure) for sleep increases. This pressure is only lessened by sleep itself.

2. **Internal biological clock**

Our internal clock, or circadian rhythm, tells us night from day and is located in the hypothalamus in the brain. It requires environmental input such as sunlight and activity to help become established and is responsible for regulating sleeping and feeding patterns, alertness, body temperature, brain activity, hormone production, urine production, cell regeneration and many other biological processes.

The two most important hormones involved in these systems are:

Melatonin. This increases in the evening, causing drowsiness and lowers the body temperature (babies do not start producing their own melatonin until around 12 weeks of age).

Cortisol. This decreases in the evening, inducing relaxation, restorative sleep, healthy digestion and immune system repair, and increases in the mornings.

In new babies there are other important contributing factors that can make babies *additionally* sleepy, over and above the norm, which include:

- **Not getting enough milk due to slow flow or low milk supply**

If a baby isn't taking enough on board, her blood-sugar level will potentially drop too low. This will make her more sleepy and so starts the cycle of feeding even less, the blood sugars dropping more and the baby getting even sleepier.

- **Jaundice**

Up to 90 per cent of newborn babies will develop jaundice to some degree in the first week of life. This is when there is a build-up of bilirubin (a waste product from the natural breakdown of old red blood cells) in a baby's system and their skin, mucous membranes and eyes take on a yellowy tinge.

It is usually harmless and will clear spontaneously within a few days or weeks. Occasionally, the level of bilirubin becomes high enough to warrant the medical treatment phototherapy (a special blue light), to prevent the very rare condition kernicterus developing, which can cause damage to the brain.

When a baby has jaundice, she can become sleepier than usual and take on less milk. This can cause the jaundice to develop further as she needs to be well hydrated to help flush out the bilirubin.*

- Infection

Often the first signs of an infection that parents and carers notice is that the baby is sleeping more than usual and feeding less. Her breathing and skin colour may also change. If you are ever worried, do not hesitate to tell your midwife or doctor. No worry is ever too small and you will never be wasting their time.

What is enough sleep?

The inconvenient (but hopefully reassuring) truth is that the answer is non-specific. 'Enough sleep' is whatever is enough for *your* baby. The range in normal is huge. Any tables purporting to tell us how much babies should sleep are generally based on opinion and/or averages. Nevertheless, on the basis that many of us are keen on numbers, I thought I'd put one of them in (adapted from the NHS Choices website) on the premise that you please promise yourself to swallow this with an enormous pinch of salt.

---

* Some breastfed babies develop 'breast milk jaundice', which results in a slightly yellow skin colour for up to a month or possibly longer. This is different to the common neonatal jaundice described above. It is seen in healthy, thriving babies and is rarely a cause for concern. However, the bilirubin levels in her blood will usually be monitored to ensure that they are within the normal range.

Age	Approx. total daytime sleep (hrs)	Total number of naps	Total night-time sleep (hrs)	Approx. total sleep in 24 hours
1 week	8	very varied	8.5	16.5
4 weeks	6–7	3–4	8–9	14–16
3 months	4–5	3	10–11	14–16
6 months	3	3	10–11	13–14
9 months	2.5	2	10–11	12.5–13.5
12 months	2.5	2	10–11	12.5–13.5

This is a very rough guide and does not indicate that anything is wrong if your baby's patterns aren't fitting in a box.

For instance, if your 3-month-old baby naps for 20–45 minutes, 3 times a day, wakes 3 times in the night and is healthy, feeding well and is generally a thriving little baby, she is fine and this is enough for her.

Likewise, if she's napping for between 1½–2 hours, twice a day, waking twice in the night and is healthy, feeding well and is generally happy, your baby is also fine. She's sleeping enough for her.

On the other hand, if she is doing either of the above but is generally grizzly, hard to settle and seems visibly tired (e.g. she's rubbing her eyes, has red eyes, is yawning and/or lethargic) then this would indicate that these figures aren't adding up to enough sleep for your baby.

Rousing a sleepy baby

If we leave an especially sleepy baby to her own devices and allow her to continue to sleep unchecked, we can miss important opportunities to feed her and help her to quickly get back on track. In these cases, it is likely that some gentle coaxing to feed, whether this be by breast, syringe, spoon, cup or bottle, will be necessary. In very occasional cases where these methods may not be enough, a baby may need extra medical help to feed. For example, this may be through a naso-gastric tube (a soft, narrow tube that goes through the nose and down into the stomach) for a short while until they are stronger again.

Ideas to help stimulate her to feed are shown in this infographic.

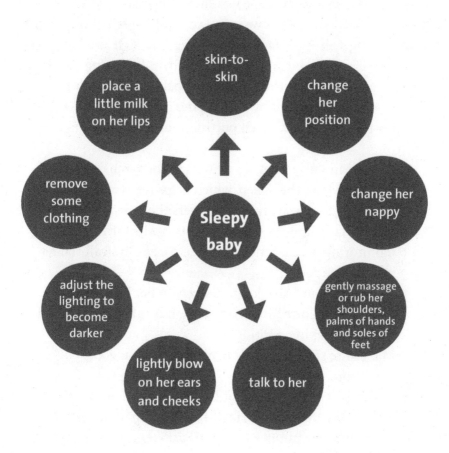

Safer sleep

Safety is paramount and, as long as safer-sleep guidelines are being followed, where exactly you choose to put your baby down for sleep depends on your preferences, space available and how you are feeding.

The guidelines exist to protect babies from sudden infant death syndrome (SIDS), also colloquially known as 'cot death', whereby a baby dies from unexplained reasons in their sleep. Although this is a horrible topic to think about, knowing how to do things safely is better than sticking our head in the sand and unwittingly doing something risky.

Around one in 3,300 babies die from SIDS each year in the UK and this number appears to be steadily falling year on year. Around 50 per cent of these babies were in a cot and the remaining 50 per cent sharing a sleep surface with a caregiver, such as a bed, armchair or sofa. The research shows that by minimising avoidable hazardous situations, the number of babies dying whilst bedsharing could be reduced by a whopping 90 per cent.

A few things to know when putting your baby to sleep:

- Babies can sense when an adult is in the same room as them whilst they sleep, which helps regulate their breathing and heart rate and lowers the risk of SIDS (particularly under 6 months). This is why relying on any monitoring device is not as protective as physically being in the same room.
- Always lie your baby down to sleep on her back (once she can roll in all directions by herself, it is safe to let her find her own sleeping position).
- Make sure the mattress is firm, clean and in good condition.
- If using blankets, put her at the bottom end of the crib or cot, so that there's no wriggle room to slip underneath.
- Keep soft toys, bumpers, sleep positioners, pillows and duvets out of the cot until she is 1 year old, as these have all been documented to be suffocation risks.
- Try to keep the room temperature between 16–20°C (or where this is impossible adjust her clothing and bedding appropriately).
- Smoking during pregnancy, and around your baby, significantly increases the risk of SIDS.
- Breastfeeding significantly reduces the risk of SIDS, with

some studies finding the difference to be as much as 50 per cent. This is thought to be because of a combination of the health-boosting properties of breast milk itself, the physical action of suckling at the breast and the amount of contact between the baby and mother.

- Around 50 per cent of babies under 3 months old share a bed with their parent at some stage in the UK. Sharing a bed with your baby becomes very risky if:

  - You or your partner have been drinking, smoking or taking any drugs/medications which can increase drowsiness
  - She gets too hot or too cold
  - She is near duvets and pillows
  - She was premature or of low birth weight (under 2.5kg)

If she is in bed with you, lie on your side to face her and place her on her back, level with your breasts. Keep any pillows or covers well away from her and keep her un-swaddled to prevent over-heating. Using a cot which

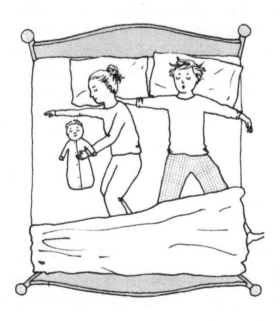

attaches on to the edge of the bed, gives some parents the reassurance that their baby is still close by whilst staying within their own sleeping space. Falling asleep lying next to your baby in a safe sleep environment in bed is *considerably safer* than falling asleep with your baby on a sofa or in an armchair, as she may become dangerously wedged on your body or between you and the furniture.

Dummy use

Some research has suggested that using a dummy for every sleep, versus occasional use of a dummy, may slightly decrease the risk of SIDS, although the reasons why are not clear. The use of a dummy, versus not using a dummy at all, does *not* affect SIDS.

Dummy use could have a negative impact on breastfeeding, particularly if one is introduced in the first 2 weeks, by interrupting establishing comfortable breastfeeding and building up a good milk supply. Sucking also releases a hormone called cholecystokinin in the baby, which leads to a feeling of satiation and sleepiness. Therefore, babies sucking frequently on a dummy may have a greater chance of missing feeds, which could lead to slow weight gain. There is an established link in the research between early dummy use and mothers stopping breastfeeding before they had originally planned. Dummies have also been linked to increased occurrences of ear, tummy and chest infections.

For these reasons, using a dummy is not an official recommendation in the UK for reducing SIDS. If you choose to introduce a dummy and are breastfeeding, try to wait until you're confident that feeding is established (usually by around 4 weeks but it may take longer) and then offer the dummy consistently at every sleep.

When a baby seems fussy and struggles to fall asleep

Inside the womb life was easy. The temperature was constantly warm, she never felt hungry, she was always held snug and her only real stimulation was the soothing sounds of your beating heart and voice, your movements and other muffled noises.

Life on the outside is tough in comparison. Everything is different and unfamiliar. Bright lights, crisp sounds, firm surfaces, space to stretch, reduced movements, a breeze in the air and feeling what it's like to be hungry. Adapting to their new environment out in the world and regaining their sense of organisation that they had in the womb can take several months or longer, a period often referred to as the 4th trimester. As a result, some babies can appear very unsettled and be awake for long periods of time, despite being tired and otherwise perfectly healthy.

As and when your baby is waking and/or isn't settling, try to interpret this behaviour as their way of communicating their needs with you and not as a form of manipulation. A mantra I love to use to explain this is: She's not *giving* you a hard time, she's *having* a hard time. This helps us to see things from her point of view and motivates us to figure out what she needs.

Cluster feeding

A classic time for things to really kick off is in the first part of the evening and night, when babies often display fussy feeding behaviour commonly known as cluster feeding. So-called fussing can be differentiated from colic (discussed later). Fussy babies may cry and often need to be rocked, carried, cuddled and constantly feed, fuss, cry, feed, fuss, cry, sleep (and so it goes on!) in ongoing bursts for several hours or more each evening. They are, more often than not, able to be soothed, are not in pain and are displaying common and expected patterns of baby behaviour. Cluster feeding can be particularly intense in the first few months and is often misinterpreted, understandably, that she is very hungry and not getting enough milk. This is rarely true unless it is going on round-the-clock and there are other true signs of low milk intake. This behaviour is much more likely down to her very new nervous system being overloaded by being out in the world and the constant on/off feeding (this can be on a bottle as well), and it's often more to do with comfort requirements rather than the need for lots of milk. The caveat here is that, particularly in the first month, any increased sucking at the breast is also her instinctual way of helping to build up a longer-term milk supply, so it's best to let her suckle at these times, rather than give a dummy for instance.

Other reasons why your baby may seek out feeding time
Outside cluster feeding, hunger in general and the other key reasons for behavioural cues covered on page 96, there are many other explanations why babies wake up and seek comfort through feeding. Most commonly these could be because she is:

- In a dirty nappy
- Too hot or too cold
- Wanting a cuddle
- Not actually tired enough
- Being annoyed by sleepwear (e.g. itchy label or a tight waistband)
- Congested in the nose
- Getting anxious about being alone (separation anxiety)
- Unwell (possibly with a bacterial or viral infection)
- In discomfort (e.g. eczema flare-up, nappy rash or threadworms)
- Intuitively picking up on physical or emotional changes at home (e.g. a parent being unwell or unhappy, baby starting childcare and so on)
- Having a spurt in her mental and physical development and her busy brain is on overdrive processing new information and learning new skills (often most noticeable in sleep around the 4-month mark)
- Finding something in the home environment that is acting as an irritant, such as paint fumes, damp or smoke
- Teething (this is at the bottom of the list as it's often blamed for sleep problems unfairly! More often,

unsettled behaviour is due to one or more of the other points listed.) Bouts of true teething pain are short-lived, if they affect your baby at all.

Or it could involve further investigating

It's 6.30pm. The evening is looming and so is the sense of foreboding that, contrary to what some of the (not so useful) books say should be happening, you've seen how your baby will almost certainly not be going down for a long peaceful sleep any time soon. She has a cry that is so intense it seems that the windows might crack. You feel helpless and heartbroken. Your beautiful baby is inconsolably writhing about, fists clenched and face puce.

If this is happening, you may be told that it's down to colic and that you just need to ride it out and do your best in the meantime to keep it together. But here's the good news – you can often do more about it.

Colic 101

First, let's make it clear that we are not talking about unsettled fussing babies. Colic is very different and is a descriptive term referring to intense and frequent bouts of *inconsolable* crying. These crying episodes often continue for at least several hours at a time and happen regularly during the first 2–3 months of life.

Figuring out what is causing a baby to cry in this way takes a bit of detective work, especially when you have already covered all the possibilities of recovering from birth, hunger, wind, sleep and stimulation. Sometimes the root cause may not ever become entirely clear and the crying may stop as suddenly as it started by around 3 months. Even so, there are other considerations to make, as follows, if your baby is very unsettled, particularly if the crying is intensifying over time and not appearing to subside by 3 months.

Temporary (or secondary) lactose intolerance

Crying may be a reaction to tummy pain, wind and diarrhoea due to a temporary intolerance to lactose. Lactase (the enzyme) is required to break down the lactose (sugar) found in both breast milk and formula. If a baby struggles to do this effectively due to some damage in the gut, the undigested lactose will ferment in the gut and cause pain. This may be caused by prematurity, a period of diarrhoea and/or vomiting, a parasitic infection, food allergy, certain medications or simply an immature digestive system. If a baby is breastfed, this should ideally continue, over and above introducing a lactose-free formula, as breast milk itself will help the gut to heal. Trialling a dairy-free maternal diet could help if cow's milk proteins have subsequently led to gut damage in the baby and temporary lactose intolerance. Chapter 6 gives you information on different formula milk options. When the gut is given the chance to heal, temporary lactose intolerance usually goes away within around 6 weeks.

Note: This is not to be confused with congenital lactase deficiency (or primary lactose intolerance from birth), which is an *extremely rare* medical emergency in babies.

Lactose overload

This is very different to, and more common than, a true intolerance to lactose (which is often over-diagnosed) but will produce similar symptoms. With lactose overload there is a normal level of lactase in the system but due to factors regarding the management of either breast and/or bottle-feeding, a baby can end up with too much lactose in the system for them to be able to digest comfortably. For example, a breastfed baby who has a poor latch or a mother who has an oversupply of milk, may take in more dilute foremilk that has a high load of lactose and slightly less fat. This combination can speed up the passage of milk through the gut (not allowing time for the lactose to be digested) and result in the baby being hungrier sooner and thus taking in more lactose, perpetuating the cycle of pain in the gut and green, frothy and explosive stools. For formula-fed babies it is possible to give them too much milk owing to the sucking reflex of the newborn and a fast flow of milk from the teat, leading to similar problems.

Gastro-oesophageal reflux disease (GORD)

First, it is very important to differentiate gastro-oesophageal reflux (GOR) from GORD. Both are commonly and confusingly referred to simply as reflux, however they are very different from one another. GOR is when some milk is regurgitated out of the stomach in small vomits (known as 'possets') or even in large vomits. Importantly, the baby is unbothered by the experience, does not appear in pain, is healthy and grows well. Around 40 per cent of babies will have GOR to a lesser or greater degree at some point. These babies are often referred to as 'happy spitters' and the problem regarded as more of a laundry issue than a medical one.

This type of reflux should not lead to medication (although often is) and can most often be minimised through winding, staying upright for around 30 minutes after feeds and effective feeding management. This means checking that breastfed babies are attached well at the breast and able to cope with the flow of milk, whilst bottle-fed babies are in an upright position with a suitable teat for feeds. Experimenting with smaller, more frequent feeds is also a handy idea. Most babies will outgrow this by 6–12 months.

GORD, on the other hand, occurs when a baby, who may or may not be vomiting (the latter is known as 'silent reflux'), cries particularly intensely during and after feeds from pain caused by the acid refluxing up from the stomach. These babies can have difficulty putting on weight, are generally unhappy most of the time, find feeding (breast and bottle) hard, and are prone to coughing and chest infections. GORD is often the symptom of something else such as a significant tongue-tie or food allergy and going on medication simply puts a plaster over the problem, rather than getting to the root of the issue. If this ever sounds like your baby, don't hesitate to go and see a health professional and put the pressure on until you feel happy that your baby is getting the help she needs.*

---

* If your baby suddenly starts vomiting regularly for no clear reason, has blood or bile-stained vomit or has any other signs of possible illness that make you feel worried, always have this checked out immediately by a doctor and do not assume that it is GOR or GORD.

If she does require medication the recommended first-line therapy in the UK is Gaviscon, followed by ranitidine and/or omeprazole if symptoms aren't improving.

> *If I had a penny for all the times I was fobbed off with the answer 'All babies spit up' when I was looking for help with my baby's reflux. It was awful for her, it was awful for us: the constant vomiting, the lack of sleep, seeing her in obvious pain, the terrifying choking episodes. We had to fight to get the GP to even listen to our concerns. In the end it was cutting out allergens that made all the difference for her.*
>
> Karen

Tongue-tie

This is covered in more detail on page 182 but is also important to mention here as a restrictive tongue-tie can cause symptoms mirroring GORD in both bottle-fed and breastfed babies. I have seen a fair few babies who are put on medication for GORD, only to discover that a tongue-tie was the root cause of the problem and, once this was resolved, the medication was unnecessary.

Cow's milk protein allergy (CMPA)

Not to be confused with lactose intolerance (which could also occur concurrently as a result of CMPA). CMPA can cause a range of symptoms along a scale of mild to severe reactions.

There are two types of CMPA, 'IgE-mediated' or 'non-IgE mediated'. IgE-mediated responses occur very quickly and may include almost immediate reactions of wheezing, swollen eyes, an itchy rash, runny noses and coughs after exposure, as well as slower and longer-lasting reactions including bloated tummies, gas and subsequent pain, diarrhoea, constipation, vomiting, GORD (as previously described), eczema, thick cradle cap and slow weight gain. More commonly, the reaction is non-IgE mediated CMPA and is often labelled as a milk intolerance. The symptoms are largely the same although tend to be of less severity and *do not* include the immediate reactions of IgE-mediated responses. It is also possible (but much more rarely) for babies to be allergic to other allergens in a mother's diet such as soya, eggs, nuts and wheat.

So, the most important question of all ... what happens next?

- Be persistent with your health professional to help you get to the root of the issue. Taking in a diary of all the crying episodes over a period of at least one week will help them see how big a deal this is for you and your baby. Better still, take in a video as it is always typical that when you are trying to convey the pain your child is in, they are on your lap smiling and cooing.
- If a health professional does suspect or diagnose an allergy, you will *hopefully* be referred for testing (if an IgE-mediated allergy is suspected), suitably advised on elimination diets (if you are breastfeeding) and prescribed any specialist milk that may be necessary if your baby takes any formula. The most common food group to eliminate first-off is dairy and this should be done for a minimum of 3 weeks. If the symptoms do not improve, other food groups may also need to be considered but always do this with professional advice.
- Take your time before spending money on colic remedies for which there is actually next to no research-based evidence to back their claims. Brand names such as Infacol and Dentinox use a substance which claims to lower the surface tension of any bubbles of air to help them join up into bigger bubbles and possibly become easier to pass, *if* this is the issue. Gripe water, which has been around for decades (and back in the day used to contain alcohol), has varying ingredients between the brands, often including dill, sugar, sodium bicarbonate and other additives. It tastes sweet, which is possibly the

main reason babies might calm down whilst having it. Colief is a lactase-based remedy available in the UK and was developed on the premise that the lactase helps to break down lactose (sugar). Again, *if* too much lactose is an issue, it might stand a small chance of helping. If you do go down the remedy route (which I'm not in the least convinced by), just try out one thing at a time, otherwise it is impossible to tell what could be helping or not.

- Gaining more attention in recent years is the possibility that probiotic drops (Lactobacillus reuteri) may reduce crying episodes for some babies. There is currently very limited evidence for their effectiveness, but results do appear to be more convincing among breastfed babies than formula-fed babies. This probiotic bacteria also occurs naturally in breast milk.
- Try the settling techniques on page 127–8.
- Always remember that this is not your fault and if you can, get help at home and hugs whenever possible.

Hunger, wind and stimulation

For all babies, regardless of whether anything out of the ordinary may be going on or not, there are three main areas to consider alongside their sleep, when helping a baby settle into life: hunger, wind and stimulation.

Consider hunger

It might seem blatantly obvious to consider hunger first, but figuring out if this is the issue or not isn't always that straightforward – especially if you are breastfeeding and can't physically see what is going in. Sometimes a baby may be hanging out at the milk bar for hours on end and still seem hungry, which could be the case if she is not actually actively 'drinking'. However, as is often the case, a baby may be getting enough milk and yet still want to be at the breast regardless. This is because breastfeeding is as much about the act as it is about the result, and a nurturing tool in the parenting toolbox to settle a baby in almost any scenario.

We will look into the specifics of how to tell if a baby is drinking well, and what to do if they're not, in the following few chapters. For now, two clear indicators for both breastfed and formula-fed babies that tell us whether things are on track are what's coming out the other end in the nappy, and the growth chart.

Nappies

Knowing what you should expect in the nappies will help you to judge whether things need to shift with their feeding. What goes in must come out after all! If not much is going in, not a whole lot is going to appear the other end. Here is a *rough* guide of what we hope to see:

	Wet nappies in 24 hours (minimum)	Dirty nappies in 24 hours
Day 1	1 (may be more if mother has received IV fluids in labour)	At least 1 (black/brown/dark green sticky meconium)
Day 2	2	At least 1 (meconium)
Day 3	3 (starting to feel heavier)	At least 1–2 (starting to turn green)
Day 4	4	At least 1–2 (green)
Day 5	5	At least 2 (green/yellow)
Day 6	6–8	More than 2 (yellow)
Weeks 1–6	6–8	More than 2 (mostly yellow)
Weeks 6+	6–8	May be less than 1 per day (mostly yellow). Poo is generally less frequent in formula-fed babies compared to breastfed babies but not always

The consistency of poo can range from very loose to solid little pellets. Loose poo, especially in breastfed babies, is very normal and mostly nothing to be alarmed about. However, if she suddenly starts to have multiple watery poos per day and you have any niggling concern that she is becoming dehydrated, always get this checked out. Likewise, if the poo is coming out in hard pellets, she could be constipated and this always warrants getting seen to. Most often it can be easily resolved without any medication after a good quality feeding assessment and advice. After 6–8 weeks, it is common for babies to go several days, or longer, without a poo. If your baby is happy, gaining weight and the poo is soft when it finally arrives, this is not a cause for concern and isn't classed as constipation.

Other things you may spot in the nappy in the very early days:

- **A small amount of blood.** Do not be alarmed! Some baby girls will have a very light bleed from their vagina at some stage in week one. It is a 'false' menstruation and is completely harmless. Many parents don't notice it as it may be in amongst the poo.
- **Tiny orange or pink crystals.** These are salt deposits in the urine and often referred to as 'brick dust'. You may only spot them once or not at all in the first few days. If you see them beyond day 4 they could be a sign that your baby isn't getting quite enough milk at that moment. Let your midwife know and ask for some help if you are breastfeeding, to check that your baby is feeding as effectively as possible.

Growth charts

Keeping an eye on the growth of a baby is an important indicator of general health and wellbeing. The centile lines used in the charts are based on the optimal growth of healthy breastfed babies and were drawn up from the measurements of thousands of children across different countries. The charts are relevant to all breastfed, formula-fed and mixed-fed babies, are suitable for all ethnic backgrounds and there are separate charts for girls, boys and babies born before 37 weeks' gestation.

There is no perfect line to aim for, since all weights, heights and head circumferences anywhere within the range of the centile lines are considered normal. The aim is for each individual baby to follow the appropriate and optimal growth that is right for them – otherwise we would all be growing up to exact clones of each other in size and shape!

You will see that there is no line to follow between birth to 2 weeks. This is intentional, given that it's normal to lose some weight after birth, before regaining it by around 2–3 weeks old. If the loss exceeds 10 per cent of the birth weight, she should be examined to check all is well and a thorough feeding assessment should be carried out.

Thereafter, babies very rarely continue to grow along the exact same points of a line every time they are checked. If there is some dipping down or jumping up going on, don't let this worry you. A useful rule of thumb is to watch that her growth is sticking to within 2 centile lines from whichever line she was born around (either higher or lower). If her growth is going outside this band (and particularly if her weight is more than 2 centiles different from her length), it would again be important to have a proper feeding assessment to see if anything is going on that can be improved and made easier. Your baby may also be referred to have a check-over with the doctor. In most cases, there are uncompli-cated and resolvable reasons for either slow or rapid weight gain.

Note: Always go to a baby clinic or GP surgery to weigh your baby. Home weighing scales are not nearly as accurate and may cause unnecessary anxiety.

Consider wind

I highly recommend bringing up the burps and working to min-imise getting windy in general. If you hear that 'breastfed babies don't need burping' kindly let it go in one ear and straight out of the other. In theory, breastfed babies are less windy than bottle-fed babies, as there is no air inside a breast to potentially suck out. Nevertheless, there are many reasons why breastfed babies may still take wind on board. Here are a few to consider:

- Any crying
- Any fussing at the breast before latching on
- A shallow latch
- A fast letdown and/or flow of milk
- A tongue-tie

If air is not sufficiently released, it will build up and, as we saw from the windy cues in the previous table, can cause significant distress. The exact causes of hiccups, a common occurrence in young babies, are not entirely understood, although it is believed that trapped wind could possibly be a contributing factor, by putting additional pressure on the diaphragm and causing it to involuntarily contract. Although hiccups are harmless and will not distress your baby, they may disturb her ability to feed effectively and settle calmly.

Tips for minimising wind:

- Burp her during and after feeds (and even sometimes before a feed starts can help if she seems fretful). Keep her in a position where her back is straight and her chin is lifted off her chest to open up the airways and make it easier for the air to escape. Use similar pressure to how you'd applaud at the end of a mediocre show (i.e. not too feathery and not too hard) and with a calm, steady heartbeat rhythm. Patting or rubbing too firmly or quickly could feel over-whelming and have the opposite effect of creating more crying and wind.
- Avoid elasticated waistbands or anything that may be tight around her tummy.
- Check you can fit a couple of fingers inside the top of the nappy.

- Provide plenty of opportunity for her to wriggle freely about unswaddled and on a safe, flat surface.
- Lie her on her tummy with some toys (or even better, you!) in front of her eye line. She may only tolerate it for a few seconds to begin with, but this will gradually build up over the weeks.*
- Aim to make time for regular breaks on long car journeys to take her out of the seat and give her a stretch.
- Try to minimise using a car seat as somewhere to put her outside travel times.
- Consider whether anything needs modifying with her feeding (this will be covered in the next two chapters).
- Massage her tummy in a clockwise motion (the direction of the movement of the gut) BUT take a class first (these are often provided free by health visiting teams) or watch a certified infant massage instructor video online as there are some precautions to take.
- Keep her upright and close to you, as often as you feel you can, especially if wind is an issue. Holding her facing into your body will allow the gentle pressure on her tummy to help relieve windy discomfort.
- For similar reasons, if you have an exercise ball at home, lie her on her tummy on the ball and, with small movements, slowly rock and roll the ball around.

There is no evidence to support the belief that gassy or spicy foods in the mother's diet cause windy problems to breastfed babies. However, some parents swear by a problematic food, so if you suspect something in particular is bothering her, keep a food and wind diary to see if you notice any patterns emerge. Always speak to a health professional before eliminating any whole food groups from your diet, which may be necessary

---

* Tummy time is safe from newborn, although always pick her up or turn her on to her back if she falls asleep in this position.

under different circumstances if something is suspected of causing an allergy.

Consider stimulation

Imagine how you feel when you've had a jam-packed, adrenaline-fuelled day. Tired but wired. When our brains are busy over-thinking it can be harder to get to sleep and once we are, the quality of our sleep can be fitful. This frequently happens to babies and can result in increased crying, fussy behaviour and more intense cluster feeding, often leading parents to assume that there is a fundamental problem with feeding when there isn't. Take a step back and see what could be happening. Even a relatively calm and sedate day can be seen as a hectic one to the eyes and ears of a new baby, and particularly so if they are recovering from a difficult birth. Are you inundated with visitors? Is her music class pretty hectic? Are you finding yourself rushing after your older children and your baby must follow suit? For any of these situations, and there could be many others, see if anything could possibly be tweaked in the short-term that could make things easier.

The name of the game in the first few months of life is to recreate a womb-like and familiar environment in order to maximise comfort, calm and security for your baby. So, in addition to feeding responsively as we've covered, some other ideas to try are:

How to create a familiar environment

What	How	Why
Co-bathing*	Get in the bath with your baby and let her snuggle on your chest. Keep her warm by slowly pouring warm water (37–38°C) on her back. She may start rooting for the breast and feed which is great!	Babies tend to feel safe and very soothed in the water, particularly when in skin contact with a parent. Keep the lights down low
Play white or pink noise	Pre-recorded noises, sound Apps, white goods in the home (e.g. washing machine)	Reminds babies of the continuous swishing sounds of your circulatory system and the heartbeat they heard in the womb
Movement and carrying	If your baby is finding it hard to be put down, finding a wrap or carrier that suits both you and your baby can be transformational	The proximity to your body, the sound of your heartbeat and your natural movement will all bring back womb-like sensations (it will also help you keep your hands free to do other things)
Rocking and patting	Slow and rhythmic	Helps to reorganise their busy brains
Parents' smell	Stuff a muslin down your front for a few hours, or use a worn cotton shirt/vest to lay out over her sheet	Babies have a strong sense of smell and get much comfort from their favourite smell – you! →

* Always make sure there is another adult nearby in case you feel dizzy or unwell whilst holding your baby in the bath. Keep her face well above the level of the water and ensure the water is not too hot.

Gently pre-warm the mattress	Hand rubbing, a warm water bottle or warmed heat pad (remove any items before placing her down)	Reduces the temperature change from being in your arms to being laid down which may startle her
Swaddling*	Loosely wrap her in a suitable swaddling blanket (if she likes it)	Helps some babies to feel secure and reduces their startle reflex
Watching the naps	Make a written or mental note of when she is sleeping, waking up and feeding	Helps to recognise any emerging patterns. For instance, if she is normally only awake comfortably for around an hour and a half but you are now in a situation 2 hours after her last nap and she is fussing, suckling very briefly at the breast and then fussing again, it may be that she's done with feeding and needs help settling for a sleep

There is some controversy that exists with swaddling because:
- Not all babies like it and some will actively become more distressed
- It is thought to increase the risk of SIDS since swaddling can put babies into a deeper sleep and increase the chance of over-heating
- If a baby is wrapped too tightly around their hips it can increase the risk of hip dysplasia ('clicky hips')

Important safe swaddling tips:
- Never use heavy blankets or cover your baby's head
- Do not swaddle to breastfeed
- Never swaddle when bed-sharing

- If your baby doesn't like it then don't pursue it
- Stop swaddling once your baby can roll (if you haven't done so already)

Slowly teaching her when day becomes night, by introducing a predictable evening routine, also undoubtedly helps to reduce fretful feeding frenzies at bedtime going forwards. Some parents start to introduce a bedtime routine from around 2 weeks, whilst others wait for another few months or even much longer.

The timings aren't the important factor when you are beginning this. It may be 6pm one evening and 8pm the next, just do it when she is ready (ideally calm and awake). The important thing here is about conditioning her to associate a specific pattern of events with winding down for the night, such as having a wash, turning the lights down, enjoying a massage with some sleepy music, dressing for bed and then having a feed.

Don't expect your baby to necessarily fall asleep at the end of it, it can take time for her to settle into the groove. If she is still up for a party, just keep things as calm as possible with lights down and quiet voices and even pop her back into the carrier, to give you some peace (or at least free hands) to eat supper. Try and turn any screens away from her face (white light from screens can inhibit the release of melatonin) and preferably stay with her in the same room where she will be spending the night.

At night time, we always fed her in a quiet, dark room. Once we realised this was better than downstairs in the lounge with the TV and lights on, everything changed! During the daytime, fresh air was always a winner. Singing helped too and these two things still seem to help and she's 2½.

Samantha

Ponder point

What have you discovered helps settle your baby? Make a brief note to help jog your memory and to serve as a guide for anyone else that may be caring for her/him.

Dreaming of a full night's sleep

There are, of course, some babies who seem to inherently know the dream. They will spontaneously start to sleep undisturbed for 6–8 hours each night (e.g. 10pm–4am or 6am) within the first 2 or 3 months and without so much as a whimper. Nevertheless, it's crucial for most parents' sanity to remember that:

1. This is very much the exception and not the rule
    and
2. Due to any of the reasons covered in this chapter, 100 per cent consistency is very rare and many babies do revert to night-time waking.

The common idea that babies should and could be sleeping through the night by 3–4 months old can be traced back to research in the 1950s. However, their definition of 'sleeping through the night' was classified as one period of only 5 hours of sleep (e.g. 11pm–4am or midnight–5am). This is far from the classic 12 hours that sleeping through the night often implies today. In addition, the context of sleep in the 1950s was very different since babies were often sleeping in separate rooms without monitors, thereby calling into question the complete accuracy of parents' recall. It is highly possible babies were waking and simply not being heard.

In 2012, a poll of nearly 11,000 parents by the website Netmums found somewhat different conclusions to the research of the 1950s. It revealed that just shy of 26 per cent of parents reported their babies had slept through at 3 months old, and 64 per cent at 12 months old. In fact, many other studies have also shown that it is entirely normal for a happy, healthy and developing baby to wake (and often have a breastfeed) once or more at night well into the *second year* of life and sometimes beyond.

Our obsession with sleeping through can also make us feel particularly crap when babies are simply responding to huge developmental changes that affect night waking, wanting to nap, waking early and so on. This is often very evident around the 4- and 8-month mark.

Does giving formula at night help a baby sleep for longer?

There isn't a straightforward yes or no answer to this one. If breastfeeding and milk production is not going so well and a baby is clearly hungry, then giving formula at night most likely would help them sleep. However, this isn't because formula is any better at doing the trick than breastfeeding per se. Research has shown that overall, breastfed and formula-fed babies have a similar number of wake-ups in the night and that breastfeeding mothers tend to fall asleep more quickly again. In addition, because it's a young baby's reflex to suck when something is in their mouth, a baby may have fed well on the breast but continue to take more milk from a bottle, despite hunger not actually being the case. This can lead to babies being overfed and *possibly* falling into a deeper sleep for slightly longer.

If you are breastfeeding (or planning on doing so) and you would rather not introduce formula as well, I hope that you will find plenty of ideas throughout this book to help maximise how well this goes for you and to help you feel supported through the night.

If you feel that your baby would benefit from a helping hand to sleep for longer periods of time but are keen to protect how breastfeeding is going, here are some suggestions for safely encouraging longer periods of sleep.

Disclaimer! *None* of these, *some* of these or *all* of these may encourage your individual baby to have longer spells of sleep. Only through experimentation will you know what the key for your baby could be.

- Adjusting the timings and length of daytime naps (for example dropping a late afternoon nap and bringing bedtime slightly forward).
- Silencing any potential sudden noises within your control, such as phones or doorbells.
- Encouraging optimal feeding during the day and before bed.
- Holding back on responding to every little noise. Wait a moment, have a peek at your baby and judge it. If we jump in too quickly we sometimes disturb what may have just been a momentary arousal and actually cause the baby to wake up more.
- Conversely, if your baby is fairly clockwork when she stirs, it's worth experimenting with pre-empting the wake-up by staying close by and resting your hand on her, or making sure that any sleepy sound cues she's used to are playing, so that she feels this sense of security as she transitions between sleep cycles and may not fully wake up.
- Only changing the nappy if it is necessary (when the skin

feels wet, is red or the baby has done a poo). If they are in an absorbent nappy, the skin feels dry and there is no nappy rash, you could leave it for now.

- If you are bottle-feeding, have some hot water prepared in an insulated flask so you aren't having to keep your baby awake for longer than necessary.
- Introducing a 'dream feed' by gently stirring the baby to feed around 3 hours after their bedtime. This could be a breastfeed, expressed-feed via bottle, or a formula-feed, depending on your feeding choices and situation. *Note: this will only make a possible difference if the reason your baby is waking is down to hunger and not one of the many other reasons for night waking.*
- Using any of the settling techniques described on page 127–8.

Night weaning

If your little one is feeding in the night and is happy and growing well, it is truly only a problem *if it's a problem for you* as her parents and never because it's an apparent problem in the eyes of anyone else. Remember: feeding is about much more than hunger. This is regardless of whether she's 4 months, 12 months or 3 years old.

If *you* feel that you need to reduce or stop any night feeds, it's most appropriate for your baby's physical and emotional development to wait until she is at least 6 months old. Always to do so as gently as possible, be sure that she's healthy and eating and drinking well during the day. The exact way about it will vary depending on her level of understanding (a 2-year-old would be very different from an 8-month-old for instance), individual needs, your family set-up, such as whether you are bed-sharing or not and whether you are breastfeeding or bottle-feeding in the night.

For under ones (since this is where we're at with this book) who have naturally become used to falling asleep whilst suckling at the breast or bottle, firstly have a think about what other sleep cues she has in addition to feeding, such as background music, a diffused essential oil, rocking, 'ssshing' and so on. Before cutting down any feeds, it really does help to have a few other cues already in place (for at least a month ideally) that you feel are more sustainable and can carry on beyond the feeding. All this helps with feelings of safety and comfort as things move on.

When it's time to start being proactive about change, be prepared to be more tired. It's not an easy pill to swallow but unfortunately it's true that making changes like this almost certainly takes more willpower and energy to see them through than sticking with the status quo. Before you fling yourself into it, talk about it with your close support system, so that you have their back-up in whatever way might help. And remember – if at any stage it just feels plain wrong, STOP! You can always come back to it if you want to.

With bottle-fed babies, try reducing the volume at each feed in small increments over a period to allow your baby to get used to the changes. For example, give 1oz less in any bottles for 4–5 nights, then decrease by a further 1oz for the next 4–5 nights, etc. If your baby still wants to drink, offer her some water, if she is over 6 months.

For breastfed babies a well-trodden method I've used with many clients are variations (depending on the family) of the following:

1. Start by waiting until she is no longer 'actively drinking' and then gently unlatch her.
2. Quickly cover your breast and lift her up into a cuddle around your neck.
3. It sometimes helps to rest one finger gently under her chin to close her mouth if she is rooting around for the breast during light sleep.
4. If she becomes upset then let her latch-on again and repeat steps 1–3.
5. Keep doing this at every night feed until she falls asleep in your arms and you can put her down –

while layering on some other sleep cues previously mentioned.

6.   Once she starts to respond to this well and quickly falls asleep in your arms (this will usually take at least 3 or 4 nights of being consistent with it), start unlatching her earlier and earlier in each feed, each time repeating steps 2–5.

7.   Only once she starts responding calmly and quickly to this (usually at least a few weeks after starting step 1), take it a step further and pick her up but do not feed her – although the extent of this will depend on her age. For example, at 8 months it's still a good plan to feed her at bedtime and make sure she has at least one more feed before midnight (if she is waking), and then perhaps not to feed her again until 5am or 6am, for example. If you feel she is thirsty you could try offering her some water in a cup. Some parents find giving water in a bottle or using a dummy helps but bear in mind that this just adds something else to have to work on further down the line. It can also help if you have a partner or willing family member or friend to take the reins for a night or two at this stage.

8.   At this point you may find that the wake-ups have reduced or that she is no longer itching to start feeding. Where to go from here depends on if she's bed-sharing, where her cot is (if she has one) and so on. If you need further individualised sleep coaching advice, check the Resources on page 285.

What to do if your baby *just won't sleep*

Sometimes you may well feel that you've ticked off every box and tried everything you feel happy with, and yet your baby Still. Won't. Sleep.

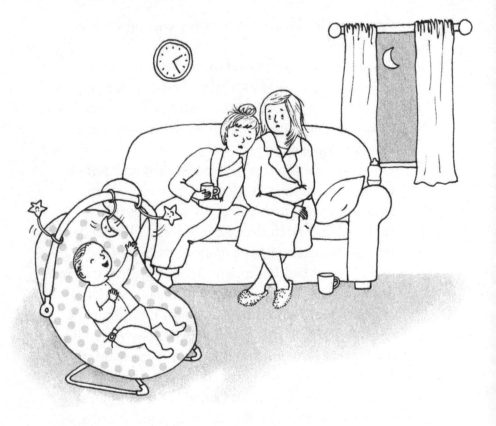

Being deprived of sleep truly is horrific. So, if and when you find yourself in the midst of it, consider the following:

- Talk to someone you trust about what's going on and how you're feeling. Whether it's a family member, friend, health visitor, GP or anyone else, sharing it will often lighten the burden. Closed online groups on Facebook and other platforms can be an invaluable source of support and place to find a virtual hug.
- Practising mindfulness techniques can do wonders in boosting energy, renewing confidence and helping you to sleep more effectively when you get the chance. The benefits of this won't only be apparent for you but can also rub off positively in settling your intuitive baby. See box opposite for Nikki's tips.

- Accept help if it is offered.
- If your instinct is telling you that your baby's interrupted sleep patterns exceed what should be considered 'normal' and her waking hours are often fussy and unsettled, then keep on seeking answers. For example, if you have a niggling doubt about a possible allergy or other concern then insist on a second opinion.
- One-to-one tailored support is nearly always better than trawling through Google. If you decide to contact an independent sleep consultant for advice, be sure to ask them about their background, philosophy and approach to ensure that you feel comfortable with their practice. Many have plenty of experience with babies but tend not to be trained in holistic assessments of babies and their families, or appreciate the full consequences of some of their advice.
- And finally, know that comparison is your toxic friend, generally serving no purpose other than to unjustly cause negative feelings in yourself. Having a baby who settles on their own and sleeps for long periods of time is never a marker of how successful you are as a parent.

Nikki's Zen Zone

Long nights can be lonely

When we're awake at night it's normal for feelings of loneliness and inadequacy to creep in. It can feel like everyone in the world is asleep, apart from you. If the nights feel like a struggle – you're not alone. And focusing on this very fact can be comforting.

Here's something to try during the night. If your little one isn't too fractious, then try and tune into the connection you're making with them. The sense of your skin touching theirs, their weight in your arms or the noises they're making. See if you can be really

→

curious about these sounds and sensations, almost as if you were experiencing them for the very first time.

If you'd like to take this a step further, you can try imagining a stream of light running between your heart and theirs. You could also lift a hand up to your heart centre and offer yourself some kind or comforting words such as 'there is warmth here now'.

Another add-on (or an alternative if the first option doesn't appeal) is to expand your awareness beyond the room you're in. Imagine the people living everyday lives in the streets and houses surrounding you. You can even imagine the people who *are* awake on the other side of the world if you like.

In doing this try to imagine the fellow parents out there awake just like you, perhaps the nurses working night shifts and other wakeful souls battling worries of their own.

Remember everyone on the earth is living with both strength and struggles – you really are not alone.

Go to: www.10ofzen.com/kindness 'In This Together' meditation.

AFFIRMATIONS

- *My baby settles into life at his/her own pace with my/our love and support*
- *I influence what I can and let go of what I can't*

5

Breastfeeding

Centuries ago, new parents would have lived near extended family who would have helped to raise each other's kids. Breastfeeding was very much on display as an everyday, visible part of life. Today we live in a different world and yet often pile the pressure on ourselves that we should simply know what to do, even if we've never seen it happening before. Some mothers and babies take to it like ducks to water, but you will also be in good company if it doesn't seem all that straightforward, especially to begin with. We've covered the whats and the whys of breastfeeding and breast milk, so this chapter will get into the nitty gritty of the *how*. We will look at:

- How breasts work
- Settling into a calm feed
- Positioning and attachment
- The ins and outs of feeding in the early days
- Specific situations whereby extra consideration might be needed, such as breastfeeding premature babies or those with additional needs
- Breastfeeding out and about
- Problem solving common (and some not so common) issues

- How breastfeeding ends, how this can feel and what to do about it

How breasts work

Breasts are simply amazing. The mammary glands inside the breast, which ultimately produce and deliver milk, start developing when we are just a 4–6-week-old embryo. This development comes to a standstill in childhood, kicking off again in adolescence and does its final bolt towards the finish line during pregnancy.

Here's how things work in a nutshell:

- During pregnancy the breasts start to make yellow colostrum (a highly concentrated version of breast milk). It's custard-thick and comes in tiny amounts. Packed full of immune factors, proteins, vitamins and minerals, it is often referred to as liquid gold and 'a baby's first immunisation'. The high levels of progesterone during pregnancy keep it in this consistency.
- The colostrum is usually all a baby will require in the early days when their tummy is just the size of a marble! This equates to around 5–7ml (or less on the first day) per feed. The first feeds are very much about quality over quantity.
- After the baby is born and the placenta is delivered, progesterone and oestrogen levels drop (although in polycystic ovary syndrome there is the possibility that oestrogen levels don't drop so much) and the process of making milk in higher volumes starts, driven by another hormone called prolactin. This is typically referred to as the milk 'coming in' from around days 2–5. I find this term misleading as it implies there is no milk before, even though we know that the colostrum is exactly what is needed to begin with. When the volume starts to increase, the colour of the milk gradually changes from

a yellow colour to creamy white. Rarely, some women notice that their milk is slightly brown. This is due to small amounts of blood from broken capillaries in the breast. It is harmless and should clear quickly. See your doctor if you are at all concerned.

- Every time the baby starts suckling at the breast, nerve endings are stimulated, causing oxytocin to be released from the brain. This contracts tiny muscles in the breast to push the milk forwards and out of the nipples. This is known as the 'letdown reflex'. Some mothers might feel a tingling sensation, increased thirst or even some pain (in the breasts and/or in the uterus), whilst others may feel nothing at all and only notice it is happening through the change in his suckling pattern.

- The more frequently a baby drinks from the breast (and/ or milk is expressed), the more the brain gets signals to keep producing milk for the future. It's a classic case of supply and demand. This means that there will most often be enough milk to feed not only one baby but also in times of greater demand for twins and even triplets too. However, if the breasts get reduced stimulation (from infrequent or ineffective suckling), particularly in the first few weeks after birth, milk production will have a much tougher time in getting set up for the future.

- If the breasts have been well stimulated, a full milk supply tends to be established by around 2–4 weeks. From this point, up until the baby is around 6 months, the amount of breast milk a baby consumes in one day is pretty much on a level playing field. The properties within breast milk itself change according to the needs of the baby, rather than the breasts constantly having to increase the volume. Between the ages of 1–6 months, the *average* volume of breast milk drunk by healthy, thriving babies in 24 hours is thought to be around 780mls (ranging from around 480ml to 1350ml).

Settling into a calm feed

I've placed this at the front of the chapter as it's a priority. How we feel, mentally and physically, going into a feed, particularly in the early weeks and months, plays out heavily on how the feed goes. The following meditation exercise isn't everyone's cup of tea, so if you feel your eyes heading skywards, don't feel in any way pushed to try it. Do exactly what is right for you.

If you have someone with you, and you fancy having a go, try out my rest and release meditation. Get yourself settled in a comfortable chair, sofa or on your bed, at a time when your baby is asleep in your arms or calmly snuggling beside you. Ask the person with you to read it out to you. They don't need to put on any strange voice; it is to be read as slowly and calmly as they can.

If you find your mind wandering off don't worry, this is completely normal, especially if it isn't something you are used to doing. Congratulate yourself for noticing the drift and bring yourself back to the meditation when you can.

Rest and release with your baby

- Start by taking three deep and conscious breaths. In through your nose and out through your mouth. Try making your outward breath a few moments longer than your inward breath.
- Notice your feet resting and notice the chair or bed underneath you holding you both. Notice the sound of my voice and any other sounds you can hear, perhaps cars, birds, talking or simply the baby's breathing.
- If you haven't done so and if you wish, allow your eyes to gently close or simply gaze down at your baby and notice how good it is to feel your eyelids becoming heavier or your gaze to be still.
- Take in another deep breath and feel your chest rising to meet

your baby. As you breathe out, imagine it to be a wave of relaxation washing over you both, each breath helping you to rest in this moment a little bit more.

- Gently take your awareness across your body and allow all these muscles to melt like butter in the sun. Notice how warm and soft your arms feel against your baby's body and how they rise and fall with each breath your baby takes.

- Now bring your awareness back to your chest, the place where we hold so many emotions, and take a moment to check in, without any judgement, and see what's there. Know that whatever you find is OK; that any thoughts you have are *just thoughts* and they don't define who you are.

- Take another few deep breaths, breathing in peace and calm and slowly breathing out any worries. Start to visualise the inside of your breasts, the incredible network of blood vessels, nerves, muscle tissue and milk ducts. See it all as if you were looking down from space at a beautiful city all lit up and sparkling at night. It's busy and connected, with traffic headlights flowing down the streets. This is you, this is your body, busily working while you rest to produce all the milk for your baby. Your body is amazing.

- Staying with this sense of just being here now resting inside your incredible body, slowly and gently come back into the room. Wriggle your fingers and toes and open your eyes when you are ready.

Once you are familiar with this exercise, you can adapt it so that it works for you wherever you are and when you are on your own. Simply take your conscious breaths, relax your eyes and work through your body, releasing any tension you find and taking a moment to check in with those incredible breasts you have right there.

Positioning and attachment (P&A)

These two words are far and away the most commonly used terms that you will hear in relation to breastfeeding. What do they mean and why are they such major players?

Positioning

Positioning refers to the physical position of your baby's body in relation to your body. Getting into a position that is effective for you and your baby is the mainstay of enjoying breastfeeding, building your supply and ensuring that your baby is drinking well.

There isn't a single position that is spot-on for everybody. We all work in different ways and what feels right for one mother will feel all fingers and thumbs for another. This also makes sense given how each mother and baby are unique in how they physically 'fit' together, given the variation in a woman's breast size, lap length, tummy shape, arm length, nipple size, shape and direction; and a baby's body size, chin shape, tongue length and mouth size. Play about with the following ideas to see what feels comfortable for you. This isn't an exhaustive list and you may well come across other positions that work for you too.

Seated or reclined positions
In seated positions, it helps to shuffle your bottom forwards a few inches, place a small cushion (or scrunched-up scarf – whatever is to hand) in the small of your back and then lean back into the chair or sofa so that your upper back and shoulders can relax. You will now be in a slightly reclined position. As you are leaning back a little, your body will provide some support for your baby. This helps him to feel relaxed, stimulates his reflexes to feed, takes some of the weight off your arms and means that you don't have to faff about too much (or at all) with cushions or pillows. Win. Once you get into the groove with this, you may well surprise yourself and find that

as well as being able to relax and put your feet up, you can also get up and about if you need to, and breastfeed whilst walking around, answering the door, eating a meal or even in the checkout queue!

These photos are just some of the ways you can hold your baby (or babies) in seated or reclined positions.

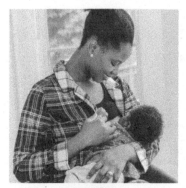

Cradle hold

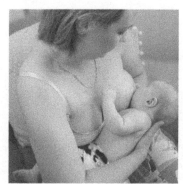

Seated cross-cradle hold

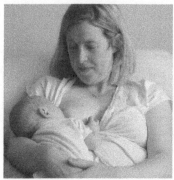

Laid-back hold (sometimes known as Biological Nurturing ®*)

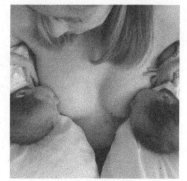

Twins feeding in a rugby or football hold

Lying positions

You can also lie on your back or side to breastfeed. Being flat on your back is possible but not necessarily the easiest, so you may prefer to prop your head and body up a little first. If you are lying on your side, following these ideas could help to make things easier:

---

* Biological Nurturing is a registered trademark owned by the Nurturing Project.

- Put a pillow behind your back can create extra comfort and support.
- If you've had a Caesarean, roll up a little blanket or find a small cushion and put it over your scar to stop any chance of little feet giving you a knock.
- Notice where your nipple (closest to the mattress) is lying. Is it touching the mattress? If so, roll back a little to lift it around an inch off the bed. This will avoid your baby having to nose-dive into the mattress to find it.

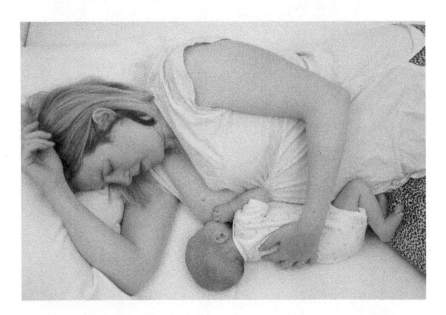

Tips for success in any position

Regardless of whether you are breastfeeding sitting at home, sprawled on a sun-lounger or hiking up a hill, there are several key principles to always have in the forefront of your mind:

- **Be aware of your body.** Take a few moments to check in with your body and notice any areas that are tense. Take a deep breath in and on the out-breath consciously let these go.

- **Have a decent 'landing pad' available.** If your clothes, bra or fingers are too close to your nipple and areola (the dark bit around the nipple), he will be unable to open his mouth wide and get a good mouthful. If you have large breasts, you may want to try rolling up a muslin or scarf and tucking it underneath your breast. This can help lift it slightly away from your chest or tummy and make it easier for you to position him.
- **Tuck the whole of his body in close to yours.** Babies gain much stability from feeling secure with their tummies and hips tucked right up against your body. If he feels all at sea with his body, he is likely to be fussier.
- **Turn the twist.** When we drink we tend to naturally adopt a position where our face is heading in the same direction as our body. Swallowing whilst looking over your shoulder is more awkward. The same goes for breastfeeding, so make sure that his hips, shoulders and face are all heading in the same direction. If he is in a bit of a twist and having to turn his head over his shoulder to reach your breasts, it will again make him fussier and drinking will be harder.
- **Keep the back of his head free.** Think about the small upward tilt we do with our chin when we drink. Babies need to get their chin off their chests as well so that they can reach up to the breast with a wide open mouth and be able to drink easily. If anything is restricting this freedom of movement, such as a hand or pillow on the back of his head, he is likely to end up head butting your breast with his mouth only partially open. This also leads to babies burying their noses in the breast. Don't worry that his head will fall off if you're not holding it! If his neck is well supported, his head will be just fine.
- **Line his body up so that your nipple lies opposite his nose and not his mouth.** Our instinct is often to line a baby up so that his mouth is right opposite the nipple.

However, what most often happens if the nipple is bang-opposite his mouth is that he won't bother to open his mouth wide, since there is no incentive for him to do so. He will then end up sucking on the nipple like a straw with a tiny little mouth. This will likely hurt for you and be ineffective at getting to the milk for him.

- When the nipple is lying opposite his nose, his rooting reflex drives him to tilt his head back a little, reach up towards the nipple, open his mouth wide and bring his tongue forward in his mouth, as the photos opposite demonstrate. This helps to ensure that he will get a good mouthful of actual breast tissue with the nipple, not just the nipple itself, which is essential for things to be comfortable for you and easy for him to feed effectively.

Attachment

Once he is all lined up, he is now ready to latch on (also known as 'attach') to the breast. Ensuring your baby is effectively attached at the breast, and isn't just nibbling or slipping on the nipple itself, can avoid and resolve most breastfeeding problems described in the Quick problem solver on page 182.

Patience at the point of latching on is paramount. As he tilts his head back, and his mouth opens wide towards the nipple, you can help him make a great connection to the breast by gently (but quickly) hugging his shoulders and upper back closer in to your body with a little pressure from your hands or forearm (remembering not to push his head forwards), depending on how you are holding him. Sometimes the window of doing this is just a SPLIT SECOND before he closes his mouth again, so keep a watchful eye, be patient and go for it without hesitation when you spy that big mouth.

A common mistake at the moment of latching is to move the breast towards the baby's mouth and physically place it into the baby's mouth, as if he were having a bottle. Doing this is another route to a painful latch with a pinched nipple, so remember to hold still and bring his body towards you, rather than you moving forwards or sideways towards him.

Depending on what position you and he are in, you may find that this 'hugging in' isn't necessary, as he could well take you by surprise and make his own way on, particularly if he is slightly on top of you and able to use his reflexes to bob his head on to the breast himself. If you were watching it all happen in slow motion, you would see the sequence of events occurring as per the following photos.

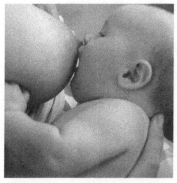

The nipple is by his nose which is stimulating his reflex to open his mouth.

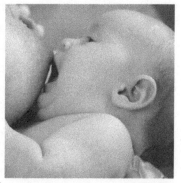

He tilts his head back, opens his mouth wider, makes contact with his chin on the breast, and with a little hug in towards his mother. Using gentle pressure on his upper back, the nipple will now enter his mouth just below his upper lip.

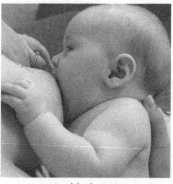

And he's on!

Signs that your baby has made a decent landing

- **You can breathe, talk, relax and even smile!** It could feel tender or even slightly painful for a few initial moments, in the early days. However, if this doesn't subside quickly after latching, or feels intensely painful *at any point*, this is your number one indicator that it's not a good latch – even if you are being told 'the latch looks great'. If it's painful, something's not right, so always ask for help to get it sorted.
- **The angle at the corners of his lower and upper lip is wide apart.** If you can't see his lips (which is a good sign!) you can gently press your boob back a little to peek. You may also see his lower lip slightly turned out, which is great.
- **His chin is wedged right in to you and there's a little gap of air by his nostrils.** This shows his chin is off his chest and he hasn't just face-planted you.
- **You can see more of the dark areola by his nose than you can by his chin.** Again, this indicates that he wasn't aiming at the centre of the dart board and has some actual breast tissue in his mouth and not just your nipple.
- **Both of his cheeks are resting equally on your breast.** His cheeks should look rounded and both be touching your breast. They should not be set back or looking sucked in. If one cheek is touching the breast and the other isn't, this could be a sign that the height of your breast versus your baby's mouth is out of sync, which can cause a drag of the breast tissue inside his mouth. He is then more likely to slip off or have a painful and/or ineffective latch. If you *do* want to hold your breast whilst he is latching and then take your hand away once he is on, always make sure that you gradually lower him down if necessary *at the same time* as your breast is making small movements, whilst you slowly release your hand. This should stop the breast slipping in his mouth.

- **He isn't making smacking or clicking sounds with his mouth.** These indicate that he hasn't got a great seal and is taking in air. Ideally, the only noise you might hear is a swallowing sound but don't panic if you don't hear this.
- **He starts to suck in a calm, rhythmic way with short pauses.** When he is actively drinking well he will take 1, 2 or 3 sucks before getting enough milk in his mouth to trigger the reflex to swallow it. When he swallows it looks like a slightly longer, slower, deeper movement of his jaw. Towards the end of a feed many babies 'flutter suck' when they get sleepy. This is gentle, faster sucking and is more for comfort than drinking milk (it's a myth that this is when a baby is gulping high-fat 'hindmilk'). If he is consistently flutter sucking throughout the feed he may not actually be drawing very much milk. This can take a bit of time to figure out so always ask for help if you need it.
- **Happy days at the end.** At the end of a feed your nipple should look round and full of colour rather than flattened or pale. Your baby, who was active at the beginning, now seems calm, settled and may even look punch drunk and conked out.

If you think the latch isn't right, take your baby off and try again. You might find that he is stuck on you like a limpet to a rock. In this case, carefully slide a clean finger into the corner of their mouth (preferably with a short nail) to break the seal first and avoid greater pain for you. In these early days, the more the two of you practise getting a great latch, rather than sitting through the pain of a pinching one, the quicker you will both get comfortable.

Sometimes, even with all the parenting will and skill in the world, a baby may simply not be in the mood or be able to efficiently 'do the textbook thing' at the point of attachment without a little more encouragement. For instance, this can happen with babies who are sleepier or have low muscle tone, or where breasts may be large, or have flat or inverted nipples. In these cases, following the 'sandwich hold' and 'nipple flipple' techniques are a top-notch way to flip your nipple towards the back of even the trickiest of mouths for attachment.

Try following these 3 steps.

1. With one hand – whichever one is free – make a 'C' shape with your thumb and fore-finger and place them on the breast. Your thumb should rest near where his nose is heading and your fingers will then be down underneath his chin. Gently compress your breast so that you are essentially making your breast into a 'sandwich' shape. Be sure to keep your fingers far enough back from your nipple so that they're not getting in the way of where his chin wants to be.

2. With your thumb still resting on your breast, use it to pull the skin back taut so that your nipple heads up and away from his mouth and the skin on the other side of your nipple bulges out towards his chin.

3. With his chin now resting on your breast and your nipple pointed up towards his forehead, roll or flip the nipple down with your thumb, past his nose and into his mouth, just under his top lip.

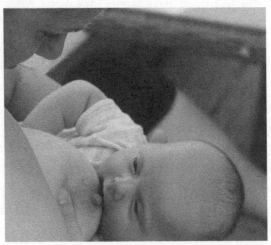

The sandwich hold and nipple flipple technique.

This can take a little practice but it is well worth sticking with it. Through trial and error you might discover your own way that works better for you, using a different combination and positioning of your fingers. As the mantra goes, do what works!

It was sore but I kept setting myself mini goals. I wanted to make it to a week, then a month and so on. The midwife who visited me on day 5 helped with her latch and I never looked back after that. It was so much more comfortable, my nipples healed and it felt more natural every day.

Bethan

The early days of breastfeeding

The first feeds (ideally kicking off in the first 'golden hour' of bonding after birth) may go on for ages or they may be short little feeds. Either are perfectly acceptable. Remember that it's not about quantity at this point but about being close to you, staying relaxed and warm. Your baby may have a fairly active period of feeding for the first 3–4 hours after birth and then have a recovery sleep. This may even last around 5 hours for some babies. As long as he fed actively beforehand and resumes business by feeding at least every 2–4 hours after this then all is generally well. There is an understandable worry about baby's blood-sugar levels dropping after birth. It is actually normal for the level to drop slightly in the first hour or two after birth and for it then to pick up again even without being fed. Colostrum (as well as skin-to-skin) is super-effective at both preventing and restoring any potential problems with low blood-sugar levels. Therefore, a little extra boost from any expressed colostrum, especially if you had gestational diabetes or are diabetic, can be very useful at this stage.

Following a Caesarean birth, it is still possible to breastfeed straight away – even in the theatre. If you've had a general anaesthetic it will take a little longer until you feel ready to hold him. Rarely, where a mother is sedated for a longer period, it may be possible for someone else to support the baby on her body to breastfeed, if she has expressly made these wishes known before.

Going into overdrive

Babies often go into fifth gear on the second or third day after birth. This does not apply to every baby; however, many babies want to feed *all the time* and may hardly sleep at all at this stage. The natural reaction is to worry that the baby is starving and simply hasn't got enough milk. This is seldom the case. What these babies are showing are instinctive desires to suck both for comfort and for bringing in your mature milk over the next few days. If your little one is up to these fun and games, know that this is common, that you are brilliant and that very soon things will start to calm down. Nevertheless, if you are at all concerned *never* hesitate to ask an experienced professional to watch a feed and help you identify when your baby is swallowing milk. If you or they still have any doubt, hand express (or use a silicone pump) to reassure yourself that your baby is getting colostrum.

WOW the milk is coming in!

On the one hand, this is an exciting time, as the reassurance of knowing that all is ticking along as it should can be huge. On the other hand, you may well have heard tales of woe from women who were struck with the sudden onset of rock hard breasts when their mature milk 'came in'. This can seriously hurt. It can also make it difficult for the baby to feed. And it doesn't help that the timing coincides with the possible baby blues, when you may have been discharged and feeling alone. Getting to the 'rock' stage is preventable in nearly every case. If it does happen, there are lots of ways to go about dealing with it rapidly to become comfortable again soon.

It is known as 'engorgement' and is generally at its peak some where between 3–5 days after birth. For most women, the breasts become full but remain squidgy enough for the baby to continue to feed efficiently and comfortably. However, in cases of extreme rock-hard-football fullness (which rarely lasts more than 24–48 hours), it can make feeding and removing milk very challenging.

This can happen for any of the following reasons:

- The baby has had long gaps between feeds (regularly feeding less often than every 2–4 hours).
- The baby may be at the breast but is not removing milk effectively (due to sleepiness, shallow latch or significant tongue-tie, for example).
- The baby is taken off the breast before they are finished.
- The baby is receiving formula or donor breast milk and is spending less time breastfeeding.
- Intravenous (IV) fluids in labour can further aggravate the situation.
- Some types of breast implants can also increase the risk of engorgement.

From this, we can see that severe engorgement is largely pre-ventable in two ways:

1. Focusing, where possible, on helping the baby to be efficient at removing milk from the breast from birth.
2. And where this isn't happening very much, or at all, regularly removing milk through expressing.

If you or your partner find themselves in the throes of engorge-ment, these tips below should quickly get things back on track.

- Lie on your back, put some vegetable-based oil on your hands and with gentle pressure, massage all around your breasts in a sweeping and circular motion from your nipples all the way up to your armpits. If you have a partner or anyone else close to you that you're happy to be involved, then all the better. Ideally keep it up for at least 20–30 minutes. Close your eyes and take this time to rest. This method helps shift excess fluid back into your lymphatic drainage system.

- Have a brief warm shower or bath, or put a warm water bottle on your breasts for no longer than a few minutes before feeding or expressing, to help the milk flow. Any longer can increase the inflammation and make things worse.
- Hand express or briefly use a silicone breast pump to begin to soften the breasts before a feed.
- Try a technique known as 'reverse-pressure softening', where you hold the tips of all your fingers in a dial around your nipple. Then press your fingertips into your breast, towards your chest wall, and hold them there for around one minute. This will help to direct some of the inflammatory fluid that has built up there away from your nipple and allow your baby to latch on a little more easily.
- Aim to remove as much milk as often as you can whilst feeding or expressing, until you feel your breasts start to soften. Don't worry about the chance of over-stimulating your breasts at this stage. The key is to get that milk shifted before it turns into a possible infection.
- During a feed gently massage your breast, this time with the direction going down towards your nipple.
- After a feed or expressing, use a cold compress on your breasts to help reduce the swelling.
- Take a full dose of an anti-inflammatory painkiller, such as ibuprofen, as required.
- The age-old cabbage leaf trick: using a knife, score the inside of a chilled, green cabbage leaf and put it inside your bra for around 20 minutes (or until it starts to wilt).

Do this no more than 3 times a day, as cabbage is thought to start reducing milk production if used for longer periods of time. Stop using it as soon as the engorgement eases off (or if you have any skin reaction).

- Be very wary of anything restrictive on your breasts, such as bras that are leaving marks on your skin, car seatbelts, lying on your side or front in bed, snoozing babies and so on.

Someone told me never to give up during the night as you always feel better about things in the morning.

Laura

Whilst any engorgement can take a day or two to subside, you may find that your breasts continue to feel heavier before a feed. By around 6–8 weeks they tend not to fill as obviously as they did before. This is nothing to worry about. It simply shows that your brain, breasts and baby are working in sync to self-regulate. Don't be tempted to wait a long time between feeds for your breasts to 'fill up'. Over time, this has the opposite effect. Your body thinks that as the milk isn't shifting anywhere particularly fast, it needn't bother making it. The more drained a breast is, the faster the rate at which it fills up again *and* with a greater concentration of higher calorie and fat-rich milk.

You might also find that you have a super-boob, with one breast that seems to have more milk than the other. It could be that you are holding your baby more on one side without realising and therefore stimulating that breast more often. This is temporary and is reversible by positioning your baby on the smaller breast first as often as possible.

Offering one or both breasts per feed

Every woman differs in how much milk her breasts can store at any one time, so ignore blanket advice to stick to one breast per feed in order to 'reach the hindmilk' (a name given to the gradually increasing concentration of higher fat milk as the breast empties). Your individual storage capacity, plus how hungry your baby is, will determine what becomes normal and necessary.

Until this becomes clear for you, it's always a good idea to try the following pattern in a feed to make sure that your baby is getting what he needs.

1. Feed from the first side until he gets agitated, falls asleep and is no longer drinking or slips off.

2. Gently wind him. This is worth trying, even if he is asleep in the early weeks (before you become familiar with what is necessary and 'normal' for him), as he may burp and start to show hunger cues again.

3. If a burp comes up relatively easily put him back on the first side, as it may well have been the trapped air that stopped him feeding. Start back at Step 1 and work through again.

4. If a burp isn't to be had, use your judgement as to whether to put him back on the first breast or try the other one. If he is already fully conked out and there's no rousing him, despite winding, and you feel that he's been drinking well, then leave him be. If the first side still feels quite full and/or he is bobbing about trying to get to it, then head back in that direction. If you can feel that he's drained your first breast comfortably and is now relaxed but showing sleepy feeding cues, he could probably do with a pick-me-up from a fresh letdown, so try him on the second side.

5. As before, feed him until he gets agitated, falls asleep and is no longer drinking or slips off.

6. Gently wind him.

7. Again, use your judgement. If the wind comes up easily and he is alert, pop him back on the same side again. If he looks very sleepy by now then leave him be.

Things will start to become clear after 2–4 weeks as to what your 'normal' feed pattern looks like and you will get a picture of your level of storage capacity. For example:

- If he mostly takes both breasts and feeds every couple of hours during the day and night, you probably have a smaller storage capacity.
- If he is fairly 50/50 about having one or both breasts and feeds roughly around 8 times in 24 hours, you probably have a moderate storage capacity.
- If he generally prefers just one breast, feeds quickly, is going for longer stretches in the day and starting to sleep longer at night, you have a larger storage capacity.

If babies are feeding effectively and according to their cues, they will thrive regardless of how much milk a mother can store in her breast at any one time. Remember this: storage capacity has nothing to do with your overall ability to make enough milk.

The length of feeds

There is no fixed time that every feed should last for (for example, at least 15 or 25 minutes) and if anyone tries to tell you otherwise, kindly let it go right over your head. Every baby feeds slightly differently depending on how hungry they are, what kind of mood they're in and how much milk the mother has stored up. Some feeds may be short and others longer. There are also a few other factors that come into play where length of feeds are concerned:

- How quickly the milk flows: ultrasounds have shown that women have very differing numbers of openings on their nipple from which the milk flows. The number you have will affect how quickly the milk comes as well as just how speedy your letdown reflex is.
- How well the baby is latched: if he isn't latched on well

then no amount of time will be long enough as he won't be able to access it very easily.

As a rule, anything ranging from around 5 to 45 minutes for one feeding session is 'normal'. Plus, remember from Chapter 4 that babies may cluster feed for longer in the early weeks and during developmental leaps.

Helping out

As a partner or anyone else supporting at home, it can feel hard to know how to help in the haze of these early days. If you can see the person you love is tired, struggling or both, it's a normal reaction to want to make things better and suggest that she either stops breastfeeding or has a break from feeding or expressing for a while. This is a big decision to take, especially during sleep deprivation, so it's worth having a chat before the baby is born about how you both might feel in this kind of scenario and what you may need from each other.

Introducing early bottles when a baby is otherwise breast-feeding well, is often the beginning of a slippery slope towards breastfeeding less frequently. If she knows that she wants to breastfeed, respecting and encouraging that decision is by far and away the most supportive and helpful thing you can do. It's not about putting any pressure on her. It's simply about listening to her and hearing what she needs without judgement. Practical things that you can do in this situation include:

- Seek out further professional help if necessary.
- Staying physically close by during feeds or expressing sessions to hug her, help her get her hair out of her face or simply stroke her arm, if that's up her street. It's the little things that count!
- Make notes of any advice given to you both so that you can recall it later.

- Take photos of her breastfeeding, particularly in positions that feel the best, so that you can help her recreate them again.
- Watch out for feeding cues.
- Bring her drinks and snacks or leave a prepared plate of food in the fridge if you need to be out, so that she can have a fuss-free grab-and-go meal.
- Prepare and maintain a comfortable 'feeding nest' with everything she may need, particularly if she'll be on her own during feeding sessions. This could include cushions, the TV remote, phone and charger, book/magazine/tablet, breast pads and nipple cream (if needed), clean muslins, a water bottle and other refreshments.
- Clean and prepare any expressing equipment that may be being used.

Don't underestimate how invaluable these little things are. You really will be making a monumental difference.

Before our baby was born I had a picture in my head that I'd be helping out by giving bottles. When I saw how much breastfeeding meant to my wife, I realised that the biggest help I could be was actually to go along with that plan and do what I could to help it work out.

Andy

What to do if your baby seems reluctant to breastfeed

If a baby simply doesn't seem up to breastfeeding when they are first born, it's not uncommon for a well-meaning 'helper' to get hands-on by pushing the baby's head on to the breast, to get things going. The thing is, babies do not like it! If someone unexpectedly pushes on the back of your head you're likely to feel fairly irritated and push your head back against the pressure. Babies generally do the same. Things can quickly turn into a battleground and babies start to instinctively feel that this is not a particularly relaxing place to hang out. As a result, they can start to get more agitated whenever they come close to the breast and appear to not want to breastfeed at all.

All this feels horrible and stressful for everyone involved. The good news is that it is an entirely reversible situation. By drawing on my acronym BASE, you can get back to basics and ride the wave of tough times such as these.

Breathe and Believe. Ask for help. Skin-to-skin. Express.

B – Breathe and Believe

Trust that this is a temporary situation and that things can and will get easier. Whilst this sounds all very well and good, it is hard to do as it's times like this that our self-critical inner voice wants to creep in and stop us in our positive tracks. Have a read of what Nikki has to say to get us through these moments.

Nikki's Zen Zone

Talk to yourself slightly differently
It's not until we stop and think about the way we're talking to ourselves that we realise we spend a disproportionate amount of time being self-critical and judging ourselves harshly. On bad days we say to ourselves things we wouldn't say to people we don't like. Sound familiar?

Self-compassion is the process of learning to offer yourself the same kindness you would readily offer your friends. Our self-critical thought processes are often well worn, so it can take time to open our hearts in this way but here's a good place to start:

Think about the kind of language you're using and see if you can do some swaps by re-framing the words:

I've got to becomes *I get to.*

Why is this happening? becomes
What is this teaching me?

I'm sorry I can't do this becomes
Thank you for being patient with me.

I'm a mess becomes *I'm human.*

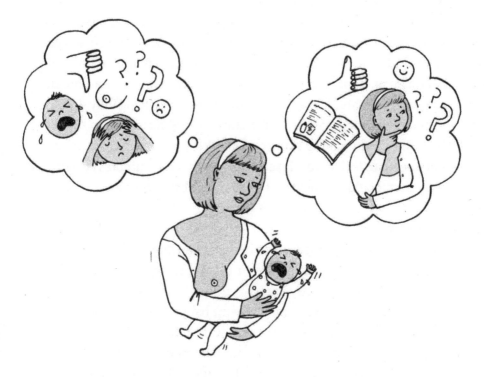

To reduce the overwhelm and help you to do this, keep things in the present. Thinking long-term – How am I ever going to be breastfeeding in 6 weeks or 6 months' time? – when you're not sure what is happening in the next hour isn't productive. Set yourself manageable goals, starting with the next few hours, then what you'd like to achieve in the next day, then the next few days, few weeks and so on. This way you can evaluate and adjust things as you go, keeping your feet on the ground and not feeling yourself spiralling off into an avoidable mental mosh pit.

A – Ask for help
As much as our knackered brains might tell us otherwise, acknowledging when help is due is a massive sign of strength and courage and *never* one that you're not being 'good enough'. The quicker you can get all the help you need the better.

S – Skin-to-skin snuggles
It may even be time to back off attempting to directly breastfeed and focus purely on happy, snuggly time together. Your baby may need space and time to 'reset' and you may be at your emotional limit and need a break from trying to breastfeed directly. We want your breasts to be a happy, safe place and not a battleground. If being fully skin-to-skin straight away feels stressful, start with him clothed and simply have his cheek making skin contact with your upper chest. As you both begin to feel more relaxed, whether this is 10 minutes or several days later, gradually increase the amount of skin contact you have.

E – Express
To keep your milk supply going in the meantime, avoid getting sore and have breast milk to give your baby, it is important to express if your baby isn't directly breastfeeding. If you are in the first few days since the birth, you can give your baby your breast milk using a 1- or 2ml syringe or you can give it directly off a spoon. If your milk has come in and the volume has increased, other options for feeding (aside from a bottle) include finger-feeding and cup-feeding, as described opposite. If you already tried colostrum harvesting during pregnancy you will be more familiar with how to hand express and may even have a little stash that can come in handy now. If not, ask your midwife to show you how.

Alternative ways of feeding expressed milk

Finger-feeding

Depending on local policy, an infant feeding specialist in the hospital, such as an IBCLC, may show you how to finger-feed your baby using a soft, narrow tube taped to your finger. One end of the tube sits in a bottle of expressed breast milk (EBM) or formula, whilst the other end lies along the end of your finger inside his mouth. Finger-feeding attempts to mimic the experience of breastfeeding by having to suck for a few seconds before they receive the milk. The baby will have control of the flow and it ensures that he has his tongue forward over his bottom gum, a wider open mouth (than on a bottle) and will keep his jaw forward, all of which are elements of learning to breastfeed.

Cup-feeding

This is another method of supplementing a baby who is not yet fully going for it on the breast but is doing *some* breastfeeding (and therefore practising a suckling motion), with EBM or formula. He is supported to sit upright and the edge of a tiny sterile cup (such as a medicine cup, shot glass or specific feeding cup for babies) is placed on his lower lip. The cup is then tilted slightly so that the milk rests on the edge of the cup and he will bring his tongue forward to lap it up like a little kitten. It's very important not to pour the milk into his mouth.

Note: Do not attempt to do either of these without professional guidance first.

Once he is calm and relaxed with skin-to-skin contact and feeding with his cheek resting on the skin of the breast, it's time to move up a gear and gently entice him to switch to breastfeeding directly if he hasn't been. Achieving this may take anything from a day to a few weeks in some cases.

1. Feed him either with the bottle, syringe or finger close to your bare breast. Or simply allow him to suck on your finger alone (with the nail facing down on their tongue).

2. After around 30 seconds (no need to be precise – it may be less or slightly more) of calm sucking, slip out the teat, syringe or finger from his mouth and quickly (but gently) turn him towards your breast and slip in the nipple (you could try using the flipple technique described on page 152).

3. If he becomes distressed, offer him back the bottle, syringe or finger straight away and try again in another 30 seconds (or so) when he is calm.

4. If things are going well, build up the frequency that you do this from several times a day to every feed, until he is directly breastfeeding again.

5. If it's not going so well, it just means taking it more slowly and gradually building up how often you try.

A note on nipple shields

If he has got used to a bottle teat and using this switching technique isn't going brilliantly, you could try using a silicone nipple shield. These have the feel of a bottle teat and a baby will often start to suckle on them without realising that they are breastfeeding. Nipple shields can also be used in times of extreme pain, especially if it feels like you have no choice but to decide between continuing breast-feeding, having a break and expressing or stopping completely.

Even though using a nipple shield can be a fantastic hack, they will not solve the underlying cause of nipple pain or latching issues and it is always worth being careful that the baby is still latching on as deeply as possible to the actual breast and not just on to the shield. Some babies will feed like a dream from a shield for months on end. However, they are an extra hassle, can impact negatively on milk supply, will reduce the likely benefit of having the baby's saliva in direct contact with the nipple and could increase the chances of poor milk drainage, so it is generally better to err on the side of caution and only use them for as short a time as possible, if you need to start with them at all.

Maximising milk supply

Parental concern around milk supply is understandably right up there as a major reason for stopping breastfeeding earlier, or starting to mix-feed with formula, when this may not have been their initial plan. Every bone in our bodies wants to nurture and protect our babies and if there's any doubt about how much milk is there, then it's totally natural to consider if an alternative plan is needed.

The very first thing with any milk supply worry is to establish whether it really *is* a fundamental problem with supply or that any concerns aren't more likely to be stemming from areas such as sleep, wind, birth history, stimulation or your own emotions (as have been covered so far in this book).

If low milk supply and subsequent slow weight gain is the concern, following these next tips may very well help things to get on track and subsequently keep you breastfeeding for as long as you wish.

Bring on the oxytocin

If you are worried about low milk supply, the chances are your oxytocin levels have taken a bashing. Aside from all the tips given in Chapter 2 on oxytocin, we should also take a leaf out of Indonesia's book (a treasure trove of massage knowledge), where they have developed the oxytocin massage. This involves a woman being massaged around the area of her fifth and sixth rib and researchers have discovered this can have profound effects on improving letdown and increasing milk supply too.

Positioning and attachment (P&A)

Having good positioning and attachment is often the biggest key to unlocking milk supply issues.

Breast compressions

During a feed, hold the breast with your hand in a C-shape by placing your thumb and forefinger on opposite sides of your nipple. When your baby starts to suck but is not drinking, squeeze your thumb and forefinger towards each other and hold this pressure (don't roll your fingers/thumb towards the nipple). Whilst held down he will start to drink again if he is still up for it. Release the squeeze only when he has stopped drinking. If after a few seconds he isn't drinking again, repeat the process. Squeeze as he is sucking but not actively drinking and swallowing (i.e. just nibbling). This helps to both maximise how much milk he is getting and also provide the stimulation your breasts need to make more.

Switch nursing

Moving from one breast to another L – R – L – R, when your baby is getting sleepy and has stopped swallowing, will often keep him more active, stimulate more letdown responses, enable him to drink more and ultimately increase the signals to your brain to up the milk production.

Expressing

It may be helpful to express after just a few feeds, or possibly as many as you can manage, over 24 hours depending on your circumstances. A technique known as 'power pumping' for 1 or 2 days can also give your milk supply a healthy kick-start, before going back to a less intense expressing schedule thereafter. There are different ways of going about power pumping. You could try expressing every hour for 5–10 minutes each time for a day. Or you could express in 3–4 hourly cycles, for 1 or 2 days including: expressing for 20 minutes, resting for 10 minutes, expressing again for 10 minutes, resting for 10 minutes and finally expressing for another 10 minutes. See page 220 for more expressing tips.

Galactagogues

These are any substances (often herbal) thought to increase milk production. However, simply because herbal remedies are 'natural' does not mean that they are entirely safe and they should always be taken with advice from a suitable professional. Although most of these remedies (which come in capsules, tinctures and teas) have not been strongly scientifically proven, there is a raft of anecdotal evidence from women themselves, who believe that they helped their milk supply in some cases. Capsules tend to have the strongest effect. The amount of active ingredient in a tea is tiny and a mother would have to be drinking gallons to really see any difference. However, if it helps with hydration and a general sense of positivity and wellbeing then this is only going to be a good thing!

Historically, fenugreek was a favourite of breastfeeding professionals. Now it's believed to decrease milk supply in a small proportion of women and is also not advised if there is any history of blood-sugar problems or asthma. Other herbs believed to have galactagogue properties are moringa (capsules made from the leaf of the moringa oleifera tree), blessed thistle (often thought to work best if taken in conjunction with fenugreek), goat's rue, spirulina, alfalfa, brewer's yeast, raspberry leaf and fennel.

Some people also believe that certain *foods* have galactagenic properties, although once again there is little to no scientific evidence to back this up. For example, eating oat-based foods every day such as porridge, flapjacks and biscuits is commonly believed to boost milk supply, along with a moderate intake of garlic and ginger. Once again, if it's a placebo, then no harm is being caused.

Finally, some prescription medications are known to help boost supply but should only be prescribed when all the standard advice isn't cutting the mustard as all medications come with the risk of side effects. For instance, domperidone can work rapidly within a few days. This should be prescribed for at least 2 weeks, at which point a mother may be able to slowly wean off it or continue it for longer if needs be. In the case of insulin resistance, such as with polycystic ovary syndrome, taking metformin or a natural alternative known as 'myo-inositol', could be beneficial to milk production.

Topping up

Often the first suggestion where low milk supply is being queried is to give the baby additional milk in a bottle. This often happens very hastily and taking some of these other steps first could boost supply enough to avoid needing to top up. Where a baby is show-ing signs of becoming (or being) dehydrated and/or significantly jaundiced, the number one priority is always to FEED him and this *could* mean topping him up, if these other strategies aren't proving enough at this point.

The assumption is sometimes that topping up means giving formula. If breast milk is available, from either expressing or from donor milk* and you would prefer to give this, then this should always be the first option. Formula is no richer or more calorific than breast milk and it simply doesn't make sense to introduce it when it's not necessary and isn't your choice.

Topping up your baby also doesn't have to be the beginning of the end for breastfeeding. Very often it is only required temporarily

---

* In the UK, hospital-based milk banks provide donor breast milk for the use of babies on neonatal units. If you are at home with your baby, you could opt for seeking out a personal, informal arrangement with a milk donor that is based on informed choice and trust. Many women doing this have had fantastic success and couldn't rate their experience more highly. However, this should always be under-taken with careful consideration and communication with the donor, as the milk is not screened for potential contamination with harmful bacteria, medications or viruses such as HIV.

and with the right support to keep building your supply and help-ing your baby to breastfeed, you may find that you can wean off the top-ups in a matter of days or weeks, if this is what you want. In other cases, either through choice or necessity, the top-ups may continue to support your whole breastfeeding journey.

Some practitioners can be quite hasty in recommending that top-ups be stopped very quickly so that the baby spends more time at the breast stimulating milk production. The idea is a good one in theory but in practice, depending on how big the top-ups have become (and particularly if they are largely or fully formula-based), this can lead to very hungry babies and stressed-out parents whilst the breasts are trying to play catch-up with the messages they are receiving. As a rough rule of thumb, it is often wise to take things gradually and reduce the top-ups by around 1oz (30ml) over a 24-hour period and keep things at this level for several days. Then, once you are confident that your baby is still as alert and producing lots of wet and dirty nappies, you can reduce them again by a further 1oz (30ml) in 24 hours for another few days and so on. This way, your body is being given the time to adjust and produce the extra milk that is required. Alternatively, you may well find that you don't need to be nearly so prescriptive as your baby does the work for you and starts to naturally become less and less interested in the bottle, as he fills up more and more at the breast.

Accepting that topping up might be necessary, if this wasn't in Plan A, can be very hard for some parents. Always know that there is no fault to lay at your feet in these situations and that gener-ally the one and only critic is your own self-critical voice. Talk to yourself as if you would to your best friend or sister in the same situation. A little bit of self-love goes a long way.

I stopped making myself feel bad about bottle-feeding alongside breastfeeding and began to see each breastfeed as the cherry on the cake.

Leanne

If you would like to, top-ups can be given using a device known as an 'at-breast supplementer', rather than from a standard bottle. These are either patented products (most widely available online and sometimes available at breastfeeding support venues) or can be made at home using a suitable feeding tube and feeding bottle or syringe. Either way, always seek professional advice before going down this route to ensure that it is safe and appropriate for you and your baby.

The at-breast supplementer

This is a way of giving a top-up to your baby at the same time as he is suckling at the breast. It involves a feeding tube resting at one end on your nipple going into his mouth, with the other end attached to or submerged in a bottle or bag of expressed milk or formula. They can be used by parents for a variety of reasons: for hypoplasia (see page 26); those who are inducing lactation or re-lactating; for transitioning a bottle-fed baby back to the breast; as a method of topping up a low milk supply or as a way of maintaining a breastfeeding relationship even where *no* breast milk is available.

Advantages
- It helps both the baby and mother to learn to breastfeed.
- They can be clamped or slid out from the baby's mouth when he is getting a natural letdown from the breast.
- It stimulates the breast to make more milk.
- It reduces the risk of the baby going off breastfeeding by not getting overly familiar with a bottle.
- It keeps up the breastfeeding relationship and the baby associates being there with comfort and feeling full.

Disadvantages
- It can be tricky and expensive to get hold of the correct feeding tubes (size Fr 5).
- It's something else to think about and have to clean and organise.
- It can be fiddly to get the hang of in the beginning.
- It won't solve issues of poor latch or sore nipples, so best to use when these have improved.

I have never been pregnant and I adopted both my children: Bill at 8 months and Elma from birth. I assumed I'd bottle-feed both babes until I realised induced lactation is possible. I have now breastfed Elma for 10 months and counting – at first people were shocked but everyone has been incredibly supportive. During our wait for Elma, I pumped for 8 hours a day, for 3 months, to stimulate milk and I took domperidone (following the Goldfarb protocol). When Elma first latched it was the most blissful thing. However, then came the bleeding nipples due to tongue-tie. We got it snipped on day 7 and it was the best thing we did. I combi-feed using the breast with an at-breast supplementer and am now using a bottle too. The supplementer was tricky to get the knack of but I'm so glad I persisted.

Penny

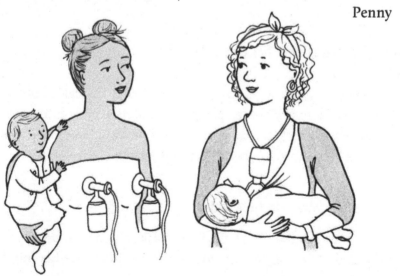

Even after a great start with milk supply, sometimes things can take a dip a few months down the road. Possible reasons for this happening include:

- Hormonal changes due to the combined contraceptive pill or a new pregnancy.
- Excessive activity or exercise level.
- Illness.
- Acute emotional shock such as a sudden bereavement or relationship breakdown.
- Changes in your daily routine such as introducing formula-feeds, consciously stretching out the time between feeds or unconsciously missing feeds because you're busy.
- Changes in your baby causing him to be more distracted or to suck with a shallow latch (which may mean he comes off after an initial letdown when the flow slows down or is simply happy suckling away but not drawing much milk).

If you're not sure what may be the cause and need more information, have a chat with your health visitor or breastfeeding specialist.

Specific situations for extra consideration

Sadly things aren't always straightforward with the health of our babies and there are some specific situations where extra consideration with breastfeeding management would be needed, as described below (please note, this is not an exhaustive list).

When your baby is in hospital

If you are unable to be with your baby, ask someone to bring you photos and videos of him and anything that may have his smell, such as a vest or blanket. These gestures can significantly help you to feel closer to your baby, boost your oxytocin levels and help with expressing your milk. If it is possible to be with him, try to express (if necessary) at his cot-side or whilst you are holding him. If he has jaundice requiring treatment, the hospital may have a bili-blanket that can be wrapped around him, so that his treatment can continue whilst he is in your arms.

Premature babies

Breast milk is often regarded as life-saving 'medicine' for very premature babies whose guts are highly sensitive and at high risk of developing a severe condition called necrotising enterocolitis (NEC). Premature babies have been known to start showing interest in the breast from as early as 28 weeks and many from 30–32 weeks. They might root, lick and do a little sucking, before their ability to coordinate and sustain a consistent suck-swallow-breathe pattern develops over the next month or so. This tends to happen more often in units that encourage skin-to-skin for as much of the time as possible. This is a method of care known as 'kangaroo mother care' (KMC) and can be used even with very premature, ventilated babies. There is strong evidence that babies' breathing, heart rate, blood pressure, temperature and blood sugars all have greater stability using KMC as often as possible, compared to when a baby is predominantly cared for in an incubator. It also supports mothers to produce more milk and encourages babies to breastfeed sooner and more effectively. If your baby is premature and you would like to be able to hold him more often than you currently are, always ask the staff if they can support you to do this.

Depending on his needs, he may start by being fed milk through a tube (usually into the nose), whilst starting to become familiar with breastfeeding. As he feeds for longer at the breast, the amount he gets in the tube will reduce until he no longer needs it. As premature babies get tired pretty easily, it is important to keep up the milk flow. When he is at the breast, using breast compressions and/or an at-breast supplementer will help him feed more actively and use less energy.

Most neonatal units should have access to donor breast milk, provided by women who produce more milk than they need at home. This milk will have been screened and pasteurised, so that it is guaranteed to be safe for your baby. If your milk supply needs some boosting from another source, donor milk is an incredible resource.

Some premature babies are prescribed milk fortifiers to potentially boost the nutritional content of their milk. These are either derived from human milk itself or from cow's milk. The jury remains out on whether these are necessary or even beneficial.

> We had a rollercoaster feeding our son born at 31 weeks. Some days were better than others but slowly, slowly it got more consistent ... expressing in the night was hard when we weren't together but I knew I wanted to do it for him and it was the one thing I could do for him that no one else could. It definitely helped me feel more connected. When he came home I was so glad I had stuck with it. He's now fully on the boob (with a little expressed every now and then – more for me than him) and such a little trooper.
>
> Jules

Babies with neurological challenges

Babies with conditions such as Down's syndrome and cerebral palsy, amongst others, often experience feeding challenges due to altered muscle tone and coordination. However, breastfeeding with the help of specialist support to show you specific ways of holding your baby (particularly in one position known as the 'dancer hold'), to build their tone and strength to feed, is very possible to all or some extent.

Cleft lip and/or palate

Providing your baby with breast milk if they have a cleft lip and/or palate is especially useful, as it tends not to aggravate the sensitive tissue in their nose and throat as much as formula milk potentially can. In addition, these babies are more prone to ear infections and breast milk will help to reduce this chance as much as possible.

With clever positioning, the breast can potentially mould to fill the gap in a cleft lip and enable direct feeding at the breast to continue. Where there is also a cleft palate, it really depends on how large and where the gap is, as to how feasible direct breastfeeding may or may not be.

Heart conditions

The physical energy it takes to breastfeed is less than it takes to bottle-feed and breastfed babies with congenital heart conditions generally have more consistent weight gain than bottle-fed babies. All these babies can tire quickly though, so feeding in response to their cues, ideally little and often, is likely to work most effectively.

If you become ill or need investigations

Most medications are compatible with breastfeeding, so if you are told that something you need to take means stopping breastfeeding or 'pumping and dumping', always err on the side of caution and check it out further. The Resources at the back of this book will help you.

Specific imaging tests such as X-rays, MRIs, ultrasounds, mammograms and CT scans do not affect breastfeeding. Contrast agent (dyes) are used in some of these tests, although there is no evidence that exposure to the tiny amount that shows up in breast milk causes toxic effects for a baby and is therefore widely felt to be safe amongst researchers. Despite this, many hospitals do have policies that advise to wait 24–48 hours as a precaution.

If the examination requires a radioactive medicine, such as for a bone, lung or thyroid scan, you will normally be advised not to breastfeed for a short period of time depending on the procedure. Most of the time the compound used is technetium (except for thyroid scans) and 75 per cent of it will be out of your body after 12 hours. Mothers expecting this type of exam can express in advance to build up a stock. If the baby has never had, or refuses, a bottle, this expressed milk could be given by cup or a product known as a 'soft-cup feeder'. Expressed milk collected in the 12 hours following the procedure can be stored and used a few days later as any radioactivity will break down and be lost.

Out and about

There is no reason to feel ashamed or apologetic when breastfeeding away from home. You are doing absolutely nothing wrong and if someone doesn't like it, they don't have to look! You are feeding and comforting your baby in the way that our human bodies were designed for. You are kicking ass.

That said, if it's not something you've experienced before, it's more than understandable if it feels fairly daunting to begin with.

I was originally self-conscious but when I realised that no one batted an eyelid it really helped. I didn't struggle at all after that. I just made sure I was wearing something that was easy to feed in, so I wasn't faffing about, and I didn't bother with covering up.

Jessica

I saw other mothers looking quite relaxed about breastfeeding in public so I thought I would be OK. When I was with other mums I was fine and felt good about doing it. However, if there were men around I felt awkward and self-conscious.

Camilla

I prefer to use a cover whilst breastfeeding out and about as it makes me feel much more comfortable. Sometimes it could be hard to get comfy but overall I've had a positive experience breastfeeding in public.

McKenzie

Have a read of these following nuggets to help boost your feeding mojo.

- **Look around.** Many people around the country will either not notice, not care (in the nicest possible way!), may smile at you, or even say something encouraging. You may be very pleasantly surprised.

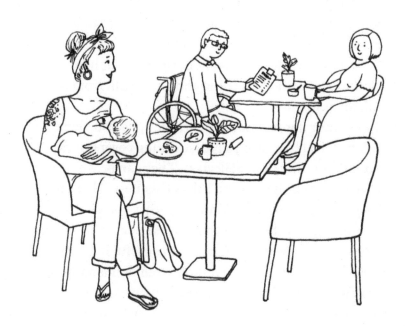

- **Take someone with you.** First time around it may be a boost to have someone alongside you. If you wanted, they could position themselves cleverly to subtly create more privacy for you and be a friendly distraction to help you to relax.

- **Prepare a comeback.** If anyone is ever rude, it reflects who *they* are, not on who *you* are, or what you are doing. Try disarming them by flashing your biggest smile, thank them for their perspective and continue doing what you're doing. By maintaining your positive stance, you will show that you have the upper hand and you will be buzzing with a sense of personal empowerment afterwards.
- **Speak the truth.** If anyone in a position of authority, such as a café manager, tries to tell you to move on, you can accurately tell them (if you are in the UK) that they can be prosecuted for their actions.
- **Think clothes.** Some mums feel happy to breastfeed by lifting their breast out over the top of their vest top, shirt or dress. However, for others, this can be a personal step too far. If you're concerned about having flesh on show, take a moment to think about how your clothes will work for feeding and practise in front of the mirror at home.
- **To cover or not to cover.** It's entirely up to you. Some mothers feel that using a breastfeeding cover draws attention rather than deflects it. They can be a hassle to use and may increases a baby's fussiness. That said, they are right for others who may otherwise choose not to breastfeed if they aren't able to use one and find they work well. They may be particularly useful if a baby is very distractible, takes a while to latch or if a mum is worried about a very fast letdown and passers-by getting a surprise spray! If you don't want to spend money on an 'official' breastfeeding cover, a muslin will generally do just as good a job.
- **Use a sling or carrier.** Granted this takes a little practice and is generally easier with older babies but if this works for you, it is a great way to feed on the go.

Periods and fertility when breastfeeding

When is it normal for periods to return?

This can happen anytime from the first few months to well into the second year or even longer. On average, the more often a mother is breastfeeding, without restrictions or mixed feeding (and especially if a baby is continuing to feed in the night), the longer periods tend to stay at bay owing to her elevated prolactin levels. Remember that it is possible to get pregnant before your periods come back as you will likely ovulate a few weeks earlier.

Is it true that breastfeeding is a contraceptive?

Exclusive breastfeeding is more than 98 per cent effective in preventing pregnancy, but ONLY if the following criteria stand:

- He is less than 6 months old
- He is being fed according to his cues during the day and the night
- He is not receiving anything else apart from breast milk
- The mother's periods have not started again

Outside these criteria anything goes, so do make sure you've thought about it if another baby isn't on the cards right now. If you're keen on going on the contraceptive pill you should be advised to use a progesterone-only pill, as oestrogen can reduce milk supply.

Being without your baby

Situations where you might find yourself away from your baby could include sudden hospitalisation, a work trip, weekend away or if he is spending time with an ex-partner. Depending on how much time you have beforehand to plan, you might want to stock-pile some expressed milk for him to have in a bottle or cup whilst you're not there. Have a look in Chapter 6 for all the information you need for this, together with travelling with breast milk and maintaining your supply whilst you are away.

Another option you may want to consider is sourcing donor breast milk or even finding another breastfeeding friend or family member to nurse your baby. Historically, this was a very common practice known as 'wet nursing' and it is often a surprise to people to hear that it regularly continues today in many cultures, including in the modern western world.

When you arrive back home, try not to be taken aback if your baby is a little off with you and it takes a few days to feel like things are back to the way they were. He may even start to wake more frequently in the night to check-in with you for a while. All this is normal and is a healthy sign of your amazing bond.

Quick problem solver

The following pages may appear a little daunting but it's important to remember that most of these problems are either truly preventable or swiftly resolvable.

Remember that how your baby is positioned and attached at the breast is *the number one* potential cause and solution for many breastfeeding issues. Rather than repetitively referring to it in the following section, I'd like to simply remind you to go over this first and foremost when looking for solutions you may be after.

Tongue-tie

Thought to be present in up to around 10 per cent of babies,* a tongue-tie could lead to attachment difficulties and thereby be a

---

* This varies across populations and the various definitions of tongue-tie used.

possible underlying factor in many of the problem areas described over the next few pages. A tongue-tie is where the stringy bit of tissue linking the underside of the tongue to the floor of the mouth is particularly short or tight and restricts the mobility of the tongue. Having a good range of motion in the tongue is essential for breastfeeding to be effective. Possible problems associated with tongue-ties (where other explanations have been ruled out) may include reduced milk supply, sore nipples, engorgement, mastitis, blocked ducts, short or very long feeds, frequent coming on and off the breast (or bottle) during a feed, large sucking blisters on the lips, excessive early weight loss, slow weight gain and difficulty controlling the milk flow. Spotting a tongue-tie is sometimes visually obvious but most often they are only picked up after a thorough digital oral examination.

Assessing for a tongue-tie is not currently part of a routine newborn check in the UK. Be conscious that most healthcare professionals, such as midwives, health visitors, GPs and paediatricians, will not have had specific training on tongue-tie assessment and diagnosis (which should never happen without taking a full breastfeeding history and assessment of a feed). This leads to both under- and over-diagnosis.

If a diagnosis of tongue-tie has been officially confirmed by a certified tongue-tie practitioner and breastfeeding is being affected as a result,* you may be advised about a frenulotomy. This is a very quick procedure to release the tie and in young babies is done without an anaesthetic, which would introduce unnecessary distress and risk. Plus, it's important that he can feed immediately after the division to relax him and get the tongue moving to stem any potential small bleed. Division of tongue-ties in young babies is offered on the NHS in most areas of the UK, if breastfeeding is being affected, although waiting lists vary. Private tongue-tie services are also available. Bodywork practitioners, such as cranial

---

* Whilst a baby may be 'diagnosed' with a tongue-tie, this does not automatically mean that it will always be the direct cause of feeding problems.

osteopaths and chiropractors, find that possible structural tension in a young baby can sometimes inhibit how freely the tongue moves and thus mimic a tongue-tie. In these cases, parents have found that breastfeeding symptoms are greatly improved with bodywork therapy and a tongue-tie division is averted.

I remember seeing his tongue-tie when he was placed on my chest for the first time. But being exhausted, I didn't follow it up until the next day when he still wasn't latching, despite numerous efforts from midwives. We found ourselves back at the hospital when he was 6 days old and a proactive consultant offered to snip it. The next day, he latched. It was incredibly emotional.

Hannah

Upper lip tie

You may also come across the term 'upper lip tie' as a breastfeeding-related issue. There is a common misunderstanding that the upper lip needs to 'flange' out on the breast in order to achieve a good latch. This is not true! In fact, an overly flanged upper lip is more often a sign of a partially open mouth achieving a shallow latch. Pouty fish lips are not what you're after. Try it out for yourself by lifting your upper lip towards your nose when your mouth is partially open. It's soft and easy to do. Now open your mouth wide and try again. The tension in the upper lip simply stops it from happening.

Whereas there is a wealth of evidence supporting the practice of an appropriate tongue-tie division, there is currently no evidence that dividing an apparent lip tie produces any benefit to breastfeeding. Despite this, it is now a common procedure in some countries such as the USA. In the UK, the NHS does not currently do these divisions for breastfeeding-related reasons.

Breastfeeding problems – causes, symptoms and suggestions

The following tables will provide you with the possible causes, the symptoms you may see and what you can do to make things better, for the four most common categories of breastfeeding problems I see in my practice:

- Painful nipples
- Painful breasts
- Fussiness or crying at the breast
- When breastfeeding is making you feel unhappy

Important note: Not all the suggestions on the following pages have had their efficacy scientifically proven beyond doubt. However, when used appropriately, they have had some positive results in my practice and/or have been reported frequently anecdotally. Always ask your health professional if you need further guidance.

Painful nipples

Possible causes	How can you tell?	What can you do about it? (in addition to P&A and TT assessment)
Nipple damage from friction	• General pain around the nipple • Redness • Red/brown blister • Cracking • Bleeding or blood in baby's spit-up (this is not harmful to the baby)	Options to treat sore nipples without cracks: • Lanolin ointment* • Breast shells (be mindful these can stimulate leaking) • Breast milk • Organic virgin coconut oil • Specific preparations with vitamin E, calendula and/or peppermint Treat cracked nipples as above. Additional options to try are: • Daily washing with mild soap • Exposure to sunlight • Hydrogel dressings/compresses • Medihoney (sterilised, medical grade honey) • Topical antibiotic cream, weak steroid cream, oral antibiotics (depending on the severity of damage and signs of infection) • Temporary use of nipple shields or expressing for 24–48 hours *Unless indicated otherwise wipe your breast clean from anything you have applied before feeding or expressing*

Milk bleb (a small white blister with milk backed up behind it caused by oversupply, pressure on the nipple, thrusht or P&A/tongue issues)	• White spot on nipple • Pin-point, needle-like pain	Apply a hot cloth, or a cotton-wool ball soaked in olive oil or coconut oil, to your nipple before trying to feed or express Then gently try and work off the thin layer of skin on the blister with your nail (a sterile needle can also be used although this should only be done with medical supervision to minimise any risk of damage or infection) Fill a cup with hot water and add a tablespoon of Epsom salts (known to be anti-inflammatory). Wait until they have dissolved and it has cooled enough to touch. Pour it into a silicone breast pump. Position the pump over the nipple with some suction. Repeat this up to 3–4 times per day Lecithin supplements may help treat and prevent stubborn plugged ducts that could be causing the blebs.
Dermatitis/ Eczema	• Redness • Blisters • Crusts • Itching • Burning	Topical corticosteroid cream and antibiotics It is very rare to only have this around one nipple at a time. Do speak to your doctor for further investigation if this is the case

* Lanolin is a naturally derived product but can still cause a red and sore reaction in some women.
† Thrush *may* be the cause if you see *more than one* milk bleb on your nipple.

Condition	Symptoms	Treatment
Vasospasm/ Raynaud's syndrome (blood vessels spasm preventing easy blood flow)	• Nipple looks white after feeds or at any time • Burning pain • Worsens in cold atmospheric conditions • Aggravated by nipple damage/ thrush infection	Keep nipple warm by covering it with a hand, towel, clothes or heat pad Massage warmed olive oil into the nipple Massage chest wall to stimulate blood supply Reduce caffeine intake Vitamin B6, magnesium and calcium supplements Prescription medication: nifedipine (may cause headaches in some women)
Nipple thrush (candida albicans)	Symptoms in mother (some or all of the following): • Burning nipple pain persisting during and after feeds, stabbing pains in the breast, painful breasts without any sore lumps or tender spots, shiny or flaking skin on the nipple or areola area	Seek help to eliminate other possibilities Best practice is to diagnose only after a positive swab test result (this is because thrush is vastly over-diagnosed and treatment given unnecessarily) If the diagnosis is made, treatment should include medication (for mother *and* baby regardless of who has symptoms), nutritional supplements (such as probiotics, zinc and B vitamins), reducing sugar and refined carbohydrate intake and careful hygiene practices at home (such as diligent hand washing, hot-washing bras, sheets and towels and regularly changing breast pads)

	• Symptoms may or may not appear on baby as well: white patches on his tongue, gums or inside of his cheeks. Oral thrush can be uncomfortable for the baby and increase their fussiness on the breast Thrush is very uncommon in the first few weeks of life, although it is more likely if the mother had thrush at the time of birth and/or has had recent antibiotics	If treatment is not working (with a positive swab) and deep breast pain is occurring, oral medication is indicated. See breast thrush on page 193)
Biting/clamping down	There's no mistaking this one – you'll feel it for sure!	As hard as it is, try not to react. If you do, your baby will find it interesting and will encourage him to try again to see if it elicits the same reaction. They are learning cause and effect! Watch his signals. It usually happens if the milk flow has slowed down and suckling is ending. Try and pre-empt it by taking him quickly off the breast Teething and boredom can be a culprit in older babies. Make sure to give him lots of opportunity to bite and chew on appropriate toys and foods, so that he doesn't feel the need to get this stimulation from your nipples!

Nipple twiddling	More common in babies older than 6 months. Whilst breastfeeding, he can find your other breast with his hand to play with. This can be sore and may feel embarrassing or annoying	Your baby is doing this for both play and comfort

If you don't want this to happen try and make your other breast as unavailable as possible

Use another distraction such as a teething/nursing necklace or give a small toy for him to play with

Gently bring the 'offending' hand up to the skin of your neck/upper chest to allow him to stroke you there |
| **Herpes of the nipple** | Painful, discrete sores around the nipple | A swab needs to be taken for viral testing. If this is herpes, your baby will need to avoid contact with this breast until the sores have healed |

Painful breasts

Possible causes	How can you tell?	What can you do about it? (in addition to P&A and TT assessment)
Engorgement	See page 154	See page 155
Mastitis (inflammation in the breast caused by milk that hasn't shifted well)	• A tender wedge or sore lump in the breast • Red streaks or a red area on the surface of the breast	The key is to keep moving the milk. Stopping feeding or going for long gaps between feeds will make it worse

Prior to moving the milk
Warmth: Bath/shower, warm gel pack or oat bag or warm water bottle (for around 5 minutes) |

• If the redness spreads, the breast feels hot, the pain is intense and you feel unwell with flu-like symptoms, it is likely to be caused by infection Important Note: on rare occasions mastitis has led to sepsis. Do not hesitate to see your doctor if you feel acutely unwell.	AND Hand massage using oil such as coconut or olive oil, in circles and strokes towards the nipple. Using an electric toothbrush or vibrator is also reported to have good results *Moving milk* Drain breast as well as possible with a deep latch and/or expressing. Position baby's chin towards the area of the lump as it will help massage it through If feeding or your normal method of expressing is not resolving it, try the technique with a silicone breast pump described for resolving milk blebs on page 187 *After moving the milk* Dunk your breast in a bowl of ice cubes or use a cold compress Rest: Go to bed – with your baby if you know how to co-sleep safely (see page 111) – eat, drink and get some help with older children or household tasks Always keep any bras or clothing loose and take anti-inflammatory pain relief (e.g. ibuprofen) if necessary

Mastitis (cont.)		Placing wet, raw potato slices on the painful area is thought to be anti-inflammatory and pain-relieving. Thinly slice a few handfuls of potatoes and put them in a bowl of water. Use a few at a time and replace when they no longer feel cool and wet (normally after around 15 minutes). Keep up the application for an hour and repeat the whole process every few hours if you wish **If after 12–24 hours of self-care the symptoms are the same or worsening then see your GP who will most likely prescribe antibiotics. If no further improvement after 48 hours ask for a swab for MRSA**
Plugged duct (a duct that has become clogged up with milk)	You can feel at least one small lump, around the size of a pea, in your breast It can happen alongside a milk bleb (page 187)	Treatment is the same as for mastitis (although plugged ducts do not normally require antibiotics) *Other points* Sunflower lecithin is a food supplement thought to make the milk 'less sticky' and reduce risk of recurrent blocked duct issues. Acupuncture has also been used with good results **If you have a persistent lump that is not going away or getting smaller after a few weeks, go and see your GP. If you need to have an ultrasound, mammogram or biopsy this does not need to get in the way of breastfeeding**

Breast abscess (a localised collection of pus, mostly caused by the bacteria S. aureus)	Early signs may have been having ongoing issues with mastitis and/or plugged ducts Diagnosis by ultrasound at a breast clinic An abscess is different from a non-painful lump that can occur during breastfeeding called a galactocele. Always check out any lingering lump with your health care professional	Breastfeeding can and should continue (even on the affected side) to prevent further problems, as milk will continue to be made in that breast and needs to be removed Treatment may involve antibiotics, repeated needle aspiration, placement of a small tube (catheter) to aid with drainage or minor surgery
Breast thrush (candida albicans)	Occasionally a thrush infection on the nipple can spread internally to the breast. This is especially likely if there has been an open wound on the nipple Women feel deep breast pain during and after feeds	All measures taken for nipple thrush should be taken plus an oral anti-fungal medication called fluconazole. It is very important to get a high enough dose to knock it on the head *Current recommendations suggest:* 400g one-off loading dose 100mg twice a day for at least 2 weeks (it can take around 5–7 days to start working even at this dose)

Mammary constriction syndrome (MCS)*	Deep breast pain associated with muscle tension in the mother. Not related to any infection	Calming techniques using breath and body relaxation
	A painful latch, or anticipation of one, can cause a mother to tense the muscles of her back, chest, neck and face. This reaction can cause constriction (squeezing) of the blood vessels serving the breast and nipple	Ask a partner, other family member or friend for a neck, shoulder and upper back massage as often as you can
	Women describe the pain differently. It can be dull or sharp, throbbing or constant, burning or itchy	Pectoral massage before each feed for around 1 minute. Massaging against the rib cage on all 4 sides of each breast: top, bottom, left and right
	It may also happen alongside vasospasm of the nipple	

* MCS was first described by Edith Kernerman IBCLC in 2013.

Fussiness or crying at the breast

Possible causes	How can you tell?	What can you do about it? (in addition to P&A and TT assessment)
Birth, wind, reflux and tiredness	See Chapters 3 and 4	See Chapters 3 and 4
Low milk supply	Fussy behaviour at the breast is only one indication of a possible issue with milk supply. Don't assume you don't have enough milk on this basis alone	Read up on these other reasons for fussy behaviour given in the table and the advice given on low milk supply on page 167
Fast milk flow	Baby may splutter, cough or gag; spit up milk often; be very windy or generally unhappy You may hear clicking or loud gulping sounds	Lying down or leaning back for feeds may help your baby have better control of the flow Wait until your letdown happens, then take him off the breast and catch the milk in a breast shell, cup or silicone pump or simply in a breast pad or towel. As things slow down, re-attach him Burp, burp and burp some more Try breastfeeding a little more frequently when your flow may be less forceful Experiment with expressing off a little milk before starting to feed. Do this with caution as you don't want to over-stimulate your breasts

Too much milk (known as 'over-supply')	Recurrent bouts of engorgement, plugged ducts and/or mastitis Excessive wind Spluttering/choking at the breast Explosive green, loose poos A feeling that you have more milk than your baby is able to drink	Have a chat with a suitable professional to ensure that this is the issue before taking any steps to reduce your milk supply Ideas to try if this is confirmed: • Peppermint (2–4 cups of tea per day) • Block feeding: Breastfeeding on one breast per feed, or for several feeds in a row before switching to the other breast (and gently expressing off the unused breast, only enough to take the edge off) • Cabbage leaves (as directed on page 156) • 1 or 2 doses of certain types of decongestant (ask your health professional) • Some women prefer to regularly express (alongside feeding) to keep their breasts comfortable and use the excess for donation milk *(Note: In the UK women are not paid for their breast milk)*
Allergy	See page 118	See page 119
Learned behaviour	See page 161 [section: What to do if your baby seems reluctant to breastfeed]	See pages 162–4

Nipple shape	Nipple shapes that *could* make things trickier may appear flat, inverted, long or particularly wide	*Flat/inverted nipples* • Try a breast pump, hand stimulation or a block of ice (briefly) on your nipple before a feed • Using the sandwich hold and nipple flipple technique is useful for flat or inverted nipples (see page 152) • Deal with any engorgement (see page 154) as this can make things harder • See a breastfeeding specialist before trying nipple shields. You may well be able to avoid it. If you do use one, make sure to be shown how to use it as effectively as possible *Large nipples* • Most babies will be able to breastfeed just fine. Premature babies may have more of a challenge breastfeeding directly until their mouth gets a little bigger. Ask for help with positioning
Nursing strike	When a baby suddenly refuses to breastfeed for no apparent reason (this is very different to a baby who is self-weaning off the breast which normally happens over a period of time)	See your GP to rule out any medical cause Keep expressing as often as you would be breastfeeding to keep up your supply and stop you getting sore

Nursing strike (cont.)	There might be a physical reason such as teething, an infection, a bunged-up nose or irritation at either too little milk or too much milk coming his way	Depending on his age, you could use a cup, bottle or soft-cup feeder if necessary. Frozen breast milk lollies are also a brilliant hack
		Try not to be tempted to force the issue, as this could make the strike last longer
	It could also be a reaction to something more subtle such as being suddenly startled during a previous feed, being distracted by a change in activity at home or even something as simple as you wearing a new perfume	Attempt to feed him when he's sleepy
		Try relaxing techniques such as co-bathing, skin-to-skin and being in a calm area
		Teething gel may work if his gums are numb
		Wear a teething/nursing necklace (made from food-grade silicone). He may like to play with this and whilst being distracted may start feeding
	Try not to panic. These are almost always temporary. Strikes can last 2–5 days, although sometimes it might go on for several weeks	Wear him in a sling or carrier with your top open to go about your business at home. The distraction of the movement and closeness to you may get him in the mood again
		An older baby may get jealous if he sees you 'breastfeeding' a toy and want to join in himself

Baby is distracted	By 3–4 months old babies start to get very interested in the world around them. This sometimes impacts on breastfeeding if they want to pull off frequently and look around	Many of the strategies for nursing strikes are also useful for distractible babies. Some babies also respond well to a nursing cover – although other babies loathe them! If things are a struggle and you are feeling isolated due to needing to feed at home, you may find it more suitable for your lifestyle to express and give him a bottle when you are out or at particular 'distractible' times you've identified

Breastfeeding is making you unhappy

Possible causes	How can you tell?	What can you do about it? (in addition to P&A and TT assessment)
Dysmorphic milk ejection reflex (D-MER)	Characterised by sudden negative feelings (such as sadness, anxiety, low mood and irritability) that start just before letdown and continue for less than a few minutes. These symptoms can feel mild to very intense	Know that this is a medical condition, not an emotional issue Track your activity, general mood and food and drink to see if you can see any pattern which may aggravate the response (e.g. caffeine, stress or dehydration) There are medications available to take on prescription for severe D-MER

Dysmorphic milk ejection reflex (D-MER) (cont.)	This is a physiological, hormonally-driven response (related to an extreme drop in dopamine). It is not psychological or related to any other breastfeeding difficulties and does not necessarily mean that the mother does not like breastfeeding or wants to stop	Some anecdotal self-help tips from women who have been through this include: • Meditation • General distraction • Magnesium spray (known for being calming and relaxing) • Vitamin B12 complex • Setting boundaries for feeding older children As a father or partner offering support, the most important thing you can do is believe what you are being told, be a non-judgemental listener and offer practical support where you can to step in and give her a break if and when she needs it
Breastfeeding aversion or agitation	Strong adverse emotional reactions to breastfeeding, whilst the baby is latched, in the absence of pain on the breast or nipple. Women describe feelings of anger, rage, agitation, irritability, itchy/skin crawling sensation and wanting to unlatch. However most want to continue breastfeeding because these negative feelings go against all their rational desires to breastfeed*	

* It happens across a spectrum of time, from specific times of the month (such as ovulation, before or during a period), to times of the day (such as at night), to during specific occasions such as extreme tiredness. There is currently a lack of research to explain why this can happen to some women but several theories include previous experience of trauma, sleep deprivation, nutritional status and hormonal regulation.

Breastfeeding burnout	You might feel irritated and stressed by the thought of carrying on breastfeeding and are thinking about stopping	Write down what is making you feel stressed to identify what your trigger points are When looking at your notes, is it breastfeeding per se, or are there other things contributing to these feelings, such as general exhaustion, money worries or other life stresses? Are you feeling any pressure from family, friends or professionals to either carry on or stop against your will? What could you do in your circumstances to help ease your trigger points? Will stopping breastfeeding make these triggers better, worse or not change them? Whether you decide to continue breastfeeding as you are, cut down or stop altogether, Chapter 2 may help with lots of tips on looking after yourself

Stopping breastfeeding

Unless there are unavoidable medical circumstances, the decision when to reduce or to stop breastfeeding entirely should always depend on when and how you want to go about it.

Weaning off the breast doesn't have to be an all-or-nothing event straight away and it also needn't be a conscious parent-led decision. If you and your baby are happy the way things are, then you may consider continuing to breastfeed until he decides himself that it's time to wind things down – he may wake up one day and simply doesn't ask for the breast again.* On the other hand, if taking charge of the weaning process is the right decision for you, it's ideal to take it as gradually as possible.

Where possible, avoid going cold turkey

This not only puts you at risk of pain, your baby will also likely be upset and confused by the sudden transition. There is also a hormonal shift at the end of breastfeeding which can leave some mothers feeling unexpectedly low for a while, even if they were happy that stopping breastfeeding was the right decision or outcome. Therefore, stopping as gradually as possible can help reduce how significant this feels. Feel comforted as well that as breast milk production decreases, the concentration of all the protective factors in the milk becomes greater, giving your baby a wonderful dollop of immunity before they say goodbye to the boob for good!

If possible, eliminate no more than one feed every 4–6 days to allow your body time to adjust. If you are not limited by time,

---

* Self-weaning is different to a nursing strike. Babies will rarely self-wean before around 18 months old and even then, it is likely due to the influence of other factors, such as being offered more solid foods or drinks in a bottle or cup. Anthropological research suggests the true natural term of breastfeeding, when left entirely in the hands of the child, to be between 2.5 and 7 years.

then it's best to try and stretch this out even further. If you need to express because your breasts begin to feel sore, take just enough milk off to relieve the pressure.

Leave their favourite feeds until last

It is much easier to stop the feeds that your little one isn't so bothered about first, which often means that sleepy feeds are the last to go. Depending on his age, you may need to replace breast-feeds with a bottle or cup of milk. If he is older than around 8 or 9 months you could offer some water and a healthy snack at some of the feedings.

Mix up the routine

If you have a favourite feeding chair, begin to sit somewhere else to give him a bottle or cup. If you lie in bed and breastfeed in the mornings, get up and have a snuggle or a play somewhere else. If someone else is on hand to help, he may respond better if they can offer some bottles in this transition phase.

Keep up lots of close physical contact

He will find weaning much easier if he knows that you are still physically present for him. Don't hold back on the kisses and cuddles. Give him lots of massages, carry him and get down on the floor to have one-to-one playtime with plenty of eye contact.

Tell him what's happening

Even young babies will benefit from open communication with you. He may not fully grasp the words but he will pick up on your gentle and understanding tone of voice. Tell him whatever you need to in simple language. For example, 'No more Mummy's milk. Mummy loves you very much.'

Don't offer, don't refuse

This is a useful strategy with older babies and children if you are not in a rush to stop. Don't sit down and offer a breastfeed. However, if he persists in asking to feed then don't refuse. In the meantime, the busier and more distracted you can keep him (plus happy with snacks and other drinks of water or milk) then the quicker he will get used to not coming to the breast.

Set limits of where, when and how much

This is another great tool to try with older ones. For example, 'You can feed when we get back home, but not here at the shops.' By the time you get home you can then use the 'don't offer, don't refuse' strategy. Also try slowly cutting back on the amount of time he spends at each feeding by gently taking him off the breast and saying to him that the milk is finished for now, before quickly distracting him with something else.

Stopping milk supply quickly

Sometimes stopping as quickly as you can is unavoidable or, if you choose not to breastfeed, the hormonal changes your body goes through after birth could still mean that your breasts may feel uncomfortably full in the first week after birth and may continue to leak a little for a while after. In these situations, using ice packs, taking anti-inflammatory pain medication and wearing extra layers (such as cotton pads in a supportive bra) to minimise any stimulation will help. You may also want or need to initially express small amounts of milk occasionally to help prevent infection.

Steer well clear of tightly binding your chest. This is dangerous advice and could lead to severe pain and possible infection. A few medications are known to suppress lactation, however some can have serious side effects and are now rarely prescribed. Some over-the-counter oral decongestants have been found to reduce milk supply in just 1 or 2 doses and are deemed safer to use. Chat to your health professional for further information.

Breastfeeding grief

Oftentimes, closing the chapter on breastfeeding marks a happy transition into another new phase of family life.

> I really loved so much about breastfeeding Connor but I knew we were both ready for it to end. I miss it sometimes but not in a sad way.
>
> Hayley

> I have zero regrets and I am so proud of myself for all the times I did manage to breastfeed her in what was quite a difficult journey.
>
> Asma

For others, it doesn't always feel like there's anything to celebrate at all. Sometimes it feels utterly crap. Devastating even. Grieving for a breastfeeding relationship that has ended, or one that was perhaps not to be, is 100 per cent real. The well-meaning, 'Come on, look at him, he's a happy and healthy baby' comments don't feel particularly welcome and can make mothers feel hurt, misunderstood and doubtful as to whether their own thoughts are important. Those thoughts *are* important and shouldn't simply be swept under the carpet.

If this is you, know that whatever it is you feel is OK. As our Zen friend Nikki reminds us *it is real to feel*. Sadness, regret, anger, guilt, heartbreak – these are just some of the emotions that breastfeeding grief can bring up and it can all hurt like mad.

Ponder point

When you have a moment of peace, fill in this exercise below. Our good old human brains often like to keep us held in the negativity zone but answering these questions can feel like shifting an unwelcome troll. It's hard to begin with but try and stick with it. There are always a ton of great things waiting to be acknowledged.

What can I celebrate about my time breastfeeding? Even if it was very brief, there are always achievements to recognise and to remember. Examples might be your time and emotional investment, the first latch, any milk you may have expressed or the comfort that being on the breast brought your baby.

What can I do now that's great? This will be very different depending on your situation. Examples might include continuing to build your connection through play, skin-to-skin, sharing baths, continuing to express some milk or have a sense of being able to reclaim your body and so on.

What do I need now to move forwards? For example, do you need to talk about this with a professional? Do you need some support with looking after older children and/or help around the home? If you have a partner, do you need them to understand how you feel?

And finally, depending on your circumstances and feelings, it may be an option if it feels right for you and your baby to 'dry breastfeed', which can also be known as 'non-nutritive sucking'. This is when a baby is suckling on the breast purely for comfort, warmth and security and is not accessing any milk. Doing this can be extremely important for some parents who dearly wish to maintain a breastfeeding relationship with their baby but do not have the milk available to meet their nutritional needs.

Re-lactation

If breastfeeding has come to an end earlier than you wanted it to, perhaps through illness or other circumstances, or if you decide at any stage that you want to give your now formula-fed baby or weaned toddler breast milk again, it is possible to bring in a milk supply and get things re-established, either partially or fully, even after a long period.* This is known as 're-lactation'. It does require a heck of a lot of determination and although it is usually more straightforward if you had a well-established milk supply previously, don't lose heart. Women who have either fully or predominantly formula-fed since the early days or weeks have shown that it can be achieved to some or all extent.

In the same way as inducing lactation, re-lactation involves expressing around the clock and possibly taking herbal supplements and/or medication (domperidone). Having plenty of skin-to-skin time and considering using an at-breast supplementer for feeds (with or without a nipple shield) are also very useful strategies. Re-lactation can be heavy-going on even the strongest of people and having lots of emotional and practical support can be crucial. Joining online groups to connect with other women in the same position to get tips and virtual hugs is hugely beneficial.

Affirmations

- I am calm with my body and my baby
- I invite in peace and let go of tension before my baby feeds
- I set manageable goals and take feeds one at a time
- I am proud of everything my body does for me and my baby
- I am not responsible for things that are outside my control
- I am proud of the mother I am

---

* It's not uncommon in parts of the world for grandmothers to re-lactate and breastfeed their grandchildren, where the mothers are ill or have died.

6

Bottle-feeding

Whether you've decided from the start that breastfeeding isn't for you, or if you'd like to now introduce bottles alongside breast-feeding, or if you have finished breastfeeding, then this chapter is for you.

In order to get going confidently with bottle-feeding, there are some key practical areas to sound out first. For that reason, this chapter will focus on:

- Choosing bottles and teats
- Sterilising and cleaning feeding equipment
- Types of breast pumps
- When and how to express
- Storing and preparing breast milk
- Introducing bottles to a breastfed baby
- Understanding different types of formula milk
- Preparing and storing formula
- How to give a bottle-feed
- Common bottle-feeding issues
- Moving from a bottle to a cup

Choosing bottles and teats

Back in the old days, choosing a bottle and teat was a very simple process. Enter the shop, pick up the bottle, pay at the till. Done. Not so much nowadays. Going into a shop, or giving it a quick Google-search, can send anyone into a spin, given the enormous range from which to choose. But does it really matter which one to go for? Are they really that different? With one quick look at the baby bottle market, it becomes very clear that their promotion is jam-packed with all sorts of claims about how their design is *the* one to go for. They know that parents' biggest concerns with bottle-feeding are around reducing wind, mini-mising interference with breastfeeding and helping a baby who is moving on from breastfeeding to accept bottles. Subsequently, we are inundated with messages about how their products can solve all these issues using emotive words such as 'natural' or 'clinically proven'.

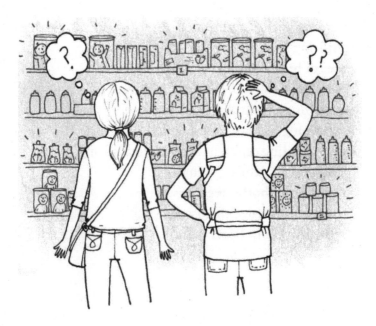

The truth is that there isn't the independent research to back up the claims and often where companies cite research papers that do, the paper trail takes you to research that does nothing of the sort. As is often the case, the fancier the product and the bigger the claim, the more money gets sucked out of your wallet when it really doesn't need to be. As we'll see later in this chapter, addressing these areas mainly comes down to how to give a bottle, rather than what type of bottle it is. Nevertheless, there are some key product considerations to be conscious of.

Material used for the bottle

It seems our ancestors were on to something when they made clay and glass baby bottles. Since the advent of plastic, billions of bottles have started filling up landfill sites. As we're becoming more conscious of our use of plastic, the glass baby bottle is making a healthy resurgence. And it's not stopping with these. Increasingly there are more stainless steel and silicone bottles available as well. The table below highlights some potential pros and cons of each type of material.

Type of material	Positives	Negatives
Plastic	Inexpensive, lightweight, easy to find and replace and are now BPA-free (a toxic chemical that has been banned in baby bottle production in the UK since 2011).	After around 6–8 weeks they start to crack, leak, become discoloured and/or smell bad. At this point they should be replaced. High turnover and inability to recycle means they quickly end up in landfill. →

		Some argue that even though they are BPA-free, there are other chemicals used in their manufacturing that should be banned as well.
Glass	No leeching of chemicals, easily recyclable, last a long time, easy to clean, many now made with a glass called borosilicate which is very robust and designed to cope with being dropped. Can also get silicone sleeves to reduce chance of breakage.	Heavier and more expensive as an initial outlay than plastic (cheaper in the long run). Not as available in shops.
Stainless steel	Lighter and less breakable than glass, easy to maintain, do not corrode, recyclable.	More expensive and heavier than plastic. Not as available in shops.
Silicone	Some consider these to be a better alternative to plastic in regards to chemicals.	Would possibly leech chemicals at very high or very low temperatures. Not as available in shops.

Size and shape of the bottle

The size of the bottle is important to consider, as the quantity of milk (particularly with formula milk) will significantly increase as your baby grows. In the first 6 weeks, she is likely to drink around 30–90mls (1–3oz) at each feed. This will then usually increase gradually to an average feed of around 90–180mls (3–6oz). It's useful to kick things off with some smaller bottles first, so that she can feed in a controlled way.

Some bottles are now being made in a 'breast-like' shape. If you like it and want to spend the money then do, but it will not be any easier or more beneficial, over and above a standard bottle shape.

Material used for the teat

Bottle teats are currently available in silicone or latex (made from natural rubber latex). Silicone is a man-made material and is transparent and odourless. Latex is derived from the sap of a specific tree. It is brown and some babies may not be fans of its initial rubbery smell (although this tends to fade after a few uses). Latex has a softer feel than silicone. A small number of babies have an allergy to latex although most brands aim to remove the allergens in the manufacturing process. Nevertheless, do be cautious if there is a family history of latex allergy.

Shape of the teat

Teats come in a huge range of shapes and sizes. The tip of the teat (the 'nipple' part) can be rounded, flattened on two sides, knobbly-looking (known as 'orthodontic'), long or short. The base of the teats come in a range of shapes from narrow to wide, or shaped to mimic the look of a breast.

As a rule, whether you are bottle-feeding a predominantly breastfed baby or one fully on bottles, I advise sticking to teats that have a medium length, rounded nipple and a medium–wide base. Look especially for teats where the angle between the nipple and the base of the teat gently slopes away and avoids a distinctive angle. These design features will help your baby to take the teat further back in her mouth and keep her mouth more widely open. This is useful for reminding a breastfed baby that she needs to have more breast in her mouth to feed effectively. It potentially benefits a fully bottle-fed baby by supporting the growth of their oral cavity in a way that enables better placement of their teeth in the future.

Whilst not everyone agrees, there is some thought that orthodontic teats teach babies to feed with their tongues pulled back. If this is the case, it's not that helpful for a breastfed baby who needs to get used to feeding with their tongue forward and flat in their mouths.

Flow of the teat

How quickly the milk comes out of the teat is the most important consideration of all. The rate of flow will vary depending on the size and number of holes in the teat. Most bottle-fed babies benefit by starting off with a slow-flow teat so that they don't become engulfed in milk, and to give them a chance at regulating both the speed at which they feed and their appetite. Indications that it is time to change the flow of the teat include spluttering or choking (go for a slower one), or if she goes from being happy feeding to starting to take much longer to feed and is getting tired or irritable (try out a faster one).

Babies with a heart condition can sometimes have a tricky time feeding from a slow-flow teat, so may benefit from moving up a gear to a slightly faster one.

If your baby has any physical additional needs, such as a cleft palate or low muscle tone, there are specialist bottles available that help babies to feed more easily in spite of their challenges.

Sterilising and cleaning

Whilst their immune systems develop, babies under 12 months are particularly susceptible to infections ranging from mild colds to more serious vomiting, diarrhoea and respiratory infections, amongst others. Bacteria (of the not so friendly kind) unfortunately feel very at home in milk and multiply quickly, providing a potentially whopping source of infection. This is particularly the case for formula milk which doesn't have the live factors of breast milk to minimise bacterial growth. This is why made-up bottles need to be chucked out if they've been sitting at room temperature for a few hours. Regardless of the type of milk, all feeding and expressing equipment should be thoroughly washed using a bottle brush in hot, soapy water or run through a dishwasher after every single use.

What happens from there is a tad confusing as, depending on where you look, you'll find different guidelines regarding the necessity for and frequency of sterilising. For example, in the UK the current advice is to wash and then sterilise all bottle-feeding equipment that has had contact with the baby after every use, until the baby is 12 months old. However, in the US, the guidance suggests running everything through a hot dishwasher, then only using a steriliser if you don't have a dishwasher and the baby is under 3 months of age, is premature or immune-compromised. Even under these circumstances they only suggest sterilising once a day. With my old nursing hat on, I tend to err on the side of caution and suggest that if you have access to sterilisation, it's only going to be a good and reassuring thing to put it to good use, particularly as dishwashers do not reach boiling point.

Sterilisation is not needed for feeding equipment for food and other drinks such as bowls, cups and spoons. They have fewer nooks and crannies for bacteria to hide and it is felt perfectly safe just to give them a thorough hot hand wash or to run them through the dishwasher. It is also currently thought necessary (in the UK) to sterilise expressing equipment once every 24 hours, although if you are in any doubt then follow the manufacturer's instructions.

Options for sterilising

There are four options for home sterilisation (unless you want to go all out and spend £300–£500 on an ultraviolet sterilising system).

1. **Cold water sterilising solution.** Equipment is fully submerged in a tub or bowl filled with water and sterilising solution, in quantities according to the manufacturer's instructions, for a minimum of 30 minutes. This solution needs to be changed every 24 hours. It's a bit smelly but inexpensive and straightforward to use. Ideally, rinse any bottle equipment after sterilising with cooled boiled water before using.

2. **Microwave steam sterilising.** This process is far quicker than cold water sterilising and does not use any chemicals. The amount of water used and exact timings will depend on the sterilising product you have and the type of microwave. Just be careful of the hot water and steam when you get it out.

3. **Electric steam sterilising.** This is the most expensive and least portable of these four options but will generally have a larger capacity to sterilise more equipment in one go and is time-efficient.

4. **Pot boiling.** A cost-free option (aside from the energy bills) is to boil the submerged equipment in a pan of boiling water for a minimum of 10 minutes. The clear downside of this method is that teats will get damaged faster so this is not a great option for frequent sterilising.

Once you have finished cleaning and/or sterilising your equipment, assemble (with your hands freshly washed) all the bits on a clean surface and then store in a clean, dry space.

Expressing to bottle-feed

There are myriad medical, social, personal, work and other lifestyle reasons why you might be expressing or using donor milk to put in a bottle. If you are expressing, you might find that simply using your own hands works best and you never need bother with a pump. If that isn't right for you, there is a range of other options available.

Try not to gauge your overall milk-making capacity by what you see coming out in a pump. Even the best pumps on the planet are not as effective or efficient at milk removal as a healthy, well-attached baby at the breast.

Always wash your hands thoroughly before starting to express.

Types of breast pumps

Type of pump	Positives	Negatives
Hospital-grade electric pumps	• Tend to have the strongest motor systems and are therefore often recommended as the best pump option for increasing milk supply • Made for multiple users by using what's termed a closed system* (a barrier between the milk and the tubing). This ensures they are safe for use between different mothers	• Fairly heavy and cumbersome • Expensive to buy • Noisy

---

* The opposite of a closed system is an open system where milk can pass into the pump tubing and potentially through to the motor and lead to a risk of mould developing within the tubing if it is not cleaned and maintained thoroughly. Open-system pumps are not made to be used between different mothers.

Type of pump	Positives	Negatives
Hospital-grade electric pumps (cont.)	• Often available for minimal rental costs (depending on need) from hospitals, children's centres or local pump rental schemes • Generally have a double-pump facility so both breasts can be expressed at the same time • Will often come with a range of breast shield sizes* (this is the conical-shaped bit that sits over your nipple) to maximise comfort and effectiveness	
Standard electric pumps (some may have battery-operated option)	• Readily available in shops • Quick to use • Ability to control suction speed and strength • Some have a double-pump facility • Most are closed-systems but double-check before multi-person use • Should have variable flange sizes but always check	• Noisy • Need to stay still and be close to a plug socket • More expensive than manual pumps • Not as effective for some mothers as hospital-grade pumps at increasing supply

* Seek advice from the product manufacturer regarding their breast shield sizing system. Generally you can tell if it is too big as the pump will easily drag your areola into the shield and it will feel uncomfortable. It is too tight if your nipple rubs the inside of the shield tunnel.

Type of pump	Positives	Negatives
Standard electric pumps (cont.)		• If borrowing or buying secondhand be aware that the motors have a shelf life. Most non hospital-grade pumps aren't designed to be used for much more than 1–2 years depending on how frequently it's in use
Battery-operated and rechargeable pumps (some may also have mains operated option)	• Modern battery-operated pumps are small, discreet and quieter than electric pumps • Able to control suction strength • Easily transportable • Can move around whilst expressing • Most are closed-systems but double-check before multi-person use	• Can be less powerful than standard electric pumps • Can be very expensive • As above re the motor • May have standard flange size
Hand pumps	• Easy to transport • Straightforward to use • Cheaper option • Quiet and discreet	• Takes physical effort and concentration as you direct the speed and strength with your hand pressing down on a lever • Suction usually not as strong as an electric pump • May only have one flange size

Type of pump	Positives	Negatives
Silicone one-piece pumps	• Small enough to be discreet in your bag • Very easy to clean and use • Cheapest of all the pump options • Requires no physical effort and (mostly) stays on hands-free • Can collect milk fairly quickly • Helpful to clear stubborn blocked ducts and engorgement	• Effectiveness varies from mother to mother. Works best when expressing or breastfeeding from the opposite breast at the same time. • They don't just 'catch the let down' so can unduly lead to over-supply • Can fall off if not attached properly or if getting full

When to express

As with selecting a pump (or variety of pumps) that work best for you, the 'rules' on when to express are again governed by what's happening in the lives of you and your baby. Here's the scoop on what could be relevant.

Exclusive expressing

Since milk storage capacity varies, expressing frequency will alter from mother to mother. Until you figure out what is necessary for you to continue to provide enough breast milk for an exclusively EBM-fed baby, express as often as she feeds throughout the day (and at night if she is night-feeding) either before, after or during her feeds. Once this is established, you could play around a little with expressing timings to see what could work best for you. For instance, an option might be to express several times close together in the mornings and then have a longer gap before expressing in another cluster later in the day. If you feel your milk supply is taking a dip then revert to what you did previously. Many mothers also choose to express at one or two extra times each day (or build up to expressing more at each session than what the baby is taking) in order to create a stand-by freezer stash.

Choosing to exclusively express for an unwell or very premature baby who is unable to breastfeed directly can become a rewarding and bonding experience during an otherwise very emotionally tough time. It is important to continue to express as frequently as you would be if she was well (at least 8–10 times in 24 hours). Where a mother expresses less often than this in the early weeks, she may well find that establishing a longer-term supply to meet her baby's growing needs further down the line becomes a lot more challenging. Natalie, who exclusively expressed for the first 12 days whilst her daughter was in intensive care, explains:

> I hand expressed for the first 2 days, with my husband catching little droplets of colostrum into a tiny syringe. On day 3, using a breast pump, I was catching 30ml from both sides each time and expressing around 10 times a day. It was incredibly uncomfortable. I had very engorged breasts, no baby to stimulate oxytocin and the baby blues made things even more emotional for me. In the end I was expressing 200ml a time and as my daughter was only 5lb 6oz, there was no way she could eat all that at that moment!
>
> Natalie

Expressing to 'top up' breastfeeding

A great supply-boosting hack is to power pump for 24–48 hours (see page 169 for more on this). Ideally, moving forward from this, a mother would then express as soon as possible after every time she breastfeeds, to maximise the increase in her supply. In the real world, this is not always feasible and if it's proving stressful, tiring and time-consuming, it may well have the opposite of the desired effect. Go for it as many times as you can, or at least after 4–6 feeds within 24 hours (including at least once or twice during the night). Waiting an hour or two after a feed to express will lessen how much is available in the breast for the next breastfeed. Although the frequency of expressing sessions is more important than the length of each session, to build up a supply, it is useful to keep expressing for a few extra minutes after no more drops are coming out. Over time this sends a clear message to your brain that what's currently happening isn't quite enough and it needs to gear up to the next level. Often this works out at around 15–20 minutes per breast but this will be different for everybody.

When you start expressing to boost your supply, don't be surprised if the amounts you are getting in the first few days are minimal or even seem to drop. This is normal and is expected. It happens because your body hasn't had the chance to act yet on the new messages your brain is getting to make more milk. Most mothers will start to see their supply increase after at least 3–4 days of additional stimulation at the breast.

Expressing to replace a regular breastfeed (for example, when going back to work)

You can choose any time of day to express that works for you, although you will probably need to express initially at the time of the feed that is being dropped to prevent issues with being uncomfortably full. If you are expressing for an evening or night-time feed, know that milk pumped in twilight/night-time hours has a higher proportion of the sleep-promoting substances tryptophan and melatonin than milk pumped in the day time.

Expressing to stockpile for going away (and being away) without your baby

When to start expressing will depend on how old your baby is and for how long you are going to be away from her. Calculate roughly how many feeds she will have in your absence and how often you can feasibly express beforehand and go from there. If you express at regular(ish) times each day, your body will start to respond by producing more milk at this time to help you build up your stored milk, without interrupting your current breastfeeding. Whilst you are away, express as often as you can to keep up your supply and avoid getting sore. If your supply does drop a little, don't worry, it will bounce back up again when you get home and back into your normal routine.

Ad hoc expressing for going out or being separated at short notice

Simple answer – just express whenever works for you. Aim to do so as soon after a breastfeed as possible and know that you can express several times in the same day if you need to and add it all together in the same bottle or storage bag.

> Being taught to hand express was amazing and the most useful thing. I had loads of milk and it was convenient for alleviating pressure when out and about, or even to quickly add some to food when weaning.
>
> Jo

Expressing the most milk you can

Even if you love everything about being a breastfeeding mum, it's unlikely that you'd look at a pump in quite the same heart-pulling way as you would your baby! Whilst this immediately puts expressing on a back pedal, the key to happy expressing is to boost your oxytocin levels. Try to harness all the oxytocin-release and calming hacks we've seen throughout the book, which you wouldn't get by simply staring down at the pump.

Aside from the more general lifestyle tips from Chapter 2, here is a quick recap of oxytocin kick-starters:

- Be comfortable and warm
- Massage the breasts with your hand
- Nipple stimulation
- Skin-to-skin (if it's feasible)
- Being close to your baby, looking at videos or pictures and smelling her worn clothes
- Body scan self-meditation (see page 142)
- Zone into the present and away from any anxious thoughts using visualisations, calming music, a funny podcast and so forth

A hack that is specific to expressing, for reasons that will become self-explanatory, has come from across the pond in the USA. You may remember the women on page 80 talking about their letdown during sex. Well, nature has a first-class provision worth noting! It's not unheard of in the US, where women are commonly back at work within 6–12 weeks of birth, to take a vibrator to work to help move things along when they are expressing. Some might cringe at the idea but hey, if it works and you want to, then go for it!

Ensuring that the whole process of expressing is pain-free is very important, so double-check the size and positioning of your breast shield, plus the settings on the pump. Some mothers have found lubricating the inside of the breast shield with a very thin smear of organic coconut oil a safe and soothing way to maximise comfort.

Finally, using any spare hands to massage and compress your breast, both whilst you are expressing and after you've finished using a pump, is a great tool for potentially getting even more milk. It's referred to as hands-on pumping.

Storing breast milk

Storing breast milk does have a small impact* on the composition of the milk itself but rest assured that if safe procedures have been followed, the milk will still be golden. Breast milk can be stored in appropriate glass or plastic containers. Steel containers are not recommended for storage as they significantly affect the breast milk composition.

Storage tips

- Remember to label each bottle or bag with the date of expression.
- Put freshly expressed milk at the bottom or at the back of your stash in the fridge or freezer, to prevent older milk getting lost and wasted.
- Allow space in your container for expansion of the milk as it freezes.
- Store in 1–3oz increments to avoid having to defrost large amounts which may potentially be wasted.
- If you are using storage bags, squeeze from the bottom of the bag and push milk slowly all the way to just shy of the top and then seal. This will remove any trapped air and will help to take up less space in the freezer.
- If you are travelling, keep the milk in a fridge, if you will be home within a few days. If you are away for longer, it would be safest to freeze the milk and then bring it home in a good quality cool box or bag with ice packs. For long journeys, some mothers have used dry ice to maintain freezer temperatures.

The Academy of Breastfeeding Medicine recommends the following timing for storage of breast milk:

---

* Some fat-soluble nutrients will stick to the inside of both glass and polypropylene containers. The most significant variations to some aspects of breast milk composition tend to happen after 3 months of freezing.

Where	How long
Room temperature (average 20°C)	4–6 hours (aim to use fresh milk over stored milk if it's available)
Ice pack in a cooler box/bag (around 15°C)	Up to 24 hours (based on one small study)
Fridge (4°C)	3–4 days (up to 8 days under very clean conditions during collection and in the fridge)
Freezer (−4°C to −20°C)	3–6 months (acceptable up to 12 months in a large freezer although quality will decrease over time)
Thawed	Keep it in the fridge and throw away 24 hours after thawing. It's not advised to re-freeze it

My wife and I are doing shared parental leave. She currently expresses at work, keeps it in the fridge for a few hours and brings it home in a cool bag. It's then refrigerated over night and I give it the following day.

Mark

Preparing stored breast milk

Thawing milk is best done slowly in the fridge or at room temperature to minimise any chance of the fat content decreasing. Where that's not an option, it can still be safely done in a bottle warmer or running the container under tepid water. Be careful not to overheat the milk as this can cause inactivation of the bioactivity in the milk and decrease the fat content. Keep well clear of the microwave. Once your baby has had her feed (and thereby introduced new bacteria to it from her mouth), the current advice is to throw away any remaining milk after 1–2 hours.

Introducing bottles to a breastfed baby

Using a bottle is not an essential rite of passage for a baby and plenty will never have one. Nonetheless, if you know that you are going to need or want to give bottles at some stage to your breast-fed baby in the first 5–6 months, it is helpful to gradually introduce an occasional one from around 6–8 weeks old. Any earlier and this could interfere with successfully establishing breastfeeding, and leaving it until 3 months or more may mean that your baby isn't so keen on the idea and takes a while to come around. If your baby is older than around 6 months then you could skip bothering with a bottle altogether and go straight on to using a cup.

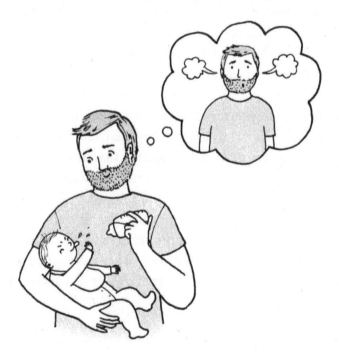

Hands down, the most crucial part of introducing a bottle is not to let it become a battle of wills and never try to force the teat into her mouth. If she associates the bottle with feeling stressed, then the whole process will take much longer. So what can you do to bottle-charm your baby? Experimentation is the name of the game. What works for one baby will be different for another.

Here are a few ideas to try:

- Let someone else try. Some babies are far more adaptable if they can't smell or see their mother.
- Try a gently sloping, medium-length teat and a medium to wide base.
- Rather than wait until she is hungry and stressed, in the hope that the bottle will get accepted, try doing it when she is sleepy or relaxed. Babies are all about feeling safe and introducing something new in an already fraught situation doesn't tend to go that well. Employ any normal settling and soothing techniques you use such as white noise, shushing, rocking or singing. These will help her to feel safe and secure and hopefully feed more calmly.
- Get her in the mood for sucking by allowing her to suck on a finger, dummy or the breast for around 30 seconds first, before quickly introducing the bottle.
- Play around with different positions and holds. She may like to be all snuggly and cosy against someone's body, or she may take it better, at least at first, if she is facing away. Using a sling and getting your salsa dancing groove on (or a gentle jiggle would suffice!) sometimes does the trick, as it feels both soothing and distracting.
- If she is the cosy type, she may respond well to having a vest or scarf that smells of her mother wrapped around the bottle and having the teat of the bottle warmed to body temperature.

If you must leave your baby before she has ever accepted a bottle, try not to freak out. If she is in the care of a loving and patient caregiver, your baby will be safe and well. She may suddenly accept the bottle for the first time. Or she may just go a few hours longer between feeds than normal and then catch up when you get home. She will be OK! If the timings necessitate that she has to take something whilst you're gone, her caregiver could always opt for a syringe, spoon, cup (if they know how to do this safely), or a product marketed as a soft cup feeder, which is a jazzed up way of spoon-feeding with more convenience and effectiveness.

> I went away for two nights when my baby was 7 months old and stressed myself silly that she wouldn't drink a thing. We offered her a bottle of pumped milk a few times a day starting 3 weeks before my trip – generally when she was sleepy – and she'd only ever drink around 1–2oz. When I was gone she was fine! She drank a bit in the bottle but actually took more from a cup and we've been going strong with a mix of the boob, bottle and cup ever since.
>
> Kym

A final idea for keeping her hydrated and calm, if she is not accepting anything else, is to leave some breast milk lollipops in the freezer.

Formula-feeding

It's not a shock to see that, as with everything in the booming baby world, there has been an explosion in the options of formula available to parents over the past few decades. It looks overwhelming, so how do you know where to start? When do you need to change? Does the price reflect their quality? Are they all necessary?

It's really simple – with a standard first milk, generally no change is necessary right the way through. If you're keen for a little more detail about what's on the shelf, then read on.

Types of formula

Marketed from birth

- **Standard powdered infant formula first milks**

This milk (marketed from birth to 6 months) is all the milk a formula-fed baby needs until they are 12 months old, unless it has been specifically recommended by a medical practitioner that she needs a different milk. As the ingredients are strictly regulated, all the first milks on the market meet legal nutritional requirements and it therefore doesn't matter whether you are buying the most expensive branded milks or the cheapest ones. The whey to casein protein ratio can differ slightly and some babies do seem to find digesting certain brands easier than others. Look for a milk where the ratio is roughly 60–40 per cent whey–casein.

Most standard first milks are based on cow's milk, with a few brands producing goat's milk-based formula as an alternative. Goat's milk formula is not suitable for babies with an allergy to cow's milk, as the make-up of the proteins are incredibly alike. Likewise, there's no point in using goat's milk formula in the hope that it will prevent a cow's milk allergy in the first place, since there is no good evidence to suggest this would be the case.

Many powdered milks are halal-approved but always check the label. Some brands also offer first milks that are organically certified.* There are also some first milks that are suitable for vegetarians because they do not contain fish oils or rennet (an animal-based enzyme). However, finding a truly vegan formula milk is currently impossible in the UK as the source of vitamin D comes from the wool of sheep.†

---

* UK regulations limit ALL formula milks to 0.01 milligrams of pesticide residue per litre. The main upsides of organic formula appear to be a lower exposure to any antibiotics which non-organic cattle may have received and a reduced impact on the environment, due to differing feeding methods of the cattle.

† A rice-based formula is sold in Europe, but it is not currently approved in the UK.

- Ready-to-feed formula (RTF)

RTF formulas are ready to pour straight into a bottle. Convenience is the obvious pull here but it's also worth weighing this up against the extra hole it'll make in your wallet and the excessive packaging. The composition of the milk is slightly different from that of its powdered milk alternative (even when it is the same branded milk) and anecdotally some parents have reported that they are convinced their baby reacts differently (namely with wind and poo). However, this is not yet backed up by any solid (ha!) research. RTF formulas are less likely to be halal-approved than their powdered milk counterparts.

- Hungry milks

The casein content is higher in these milks, with the theory (which is not backed up by good science) that it keeps babies full for longer. Although it sounds tempting, casein is harder to digest and it puts a baby's digestive system under more pressure. There is also a known link between high protein diets in small babies and health-associated issues with obesity later down the line. For these reasons, no organisation currently recommends using this type of milk.

- Comfort milks

This type of milk is based on the premise that if the protein is already partly broken down, it will be easier to digest and therefore reduce the chances of colicky episodes and constipation. However, once again (there's a theme!), there is no steady evidence to support this. There is also no evidence that these milks will prevent a milk allergy and shouldn't be used for babies who have a diagnosed cow's milk allergy. Lactose content is reduced in these milks and replaced by glucose syrup.

- Anti-reflux milks

Using thickeners such as potato starch or carob bean gum, these products aim to help milk stay where it should and not make a messy reappearance. Anti-reflux formulas (for reasons I can't fathom) can side-step infant formula regulations in the UK and will not get to the root of what may be causing any true reflux problems, so should ideally only be used with professional guidance. A common worry about these milks is that the instructions recommend making them up with the water at a lower temperature than with standard milks, to prevent the heat causing lumpiness and negatively affecting components of the milk. Powdered milks *of any kind* are not sterile products, and adding cooler water will not kill off potential bacteria that could be lurking around, so this is worth considering before deciding to use these milks.

- **Soya-based milks**

Although soya-based formula is available from birth it is generally not recommended in the UK for babies under 6 months, for the following reasons:

- The carbohydrate source is glucose.
- The use of these milks as an alternative where there is cow's milk allergy doesn't stack up, as a significant number of babies with cow's milk allergy will also have an issue with soya.
- There is a worry about phytoestrogens in soya mimicking sex hormones in the body and potentially causing earlier signs of puberty.

Depending on which side of the fence professionals tend to sit, the opinions on how significant the hormonal effects are of giving soya to young babies vary wildly. A big factor to consider is that since milk should be the *only* form of food for a baby under 6 months, the daily concentration of soya they would be receiving from milk is far higher than an older baby or child who is also having solid foods. Vegetarian and vegan families who are mixed-feeding (breast and formula) or fully formula-feeding, often opt for soya to avoid the use of fish oils and rennet. Some parents also choose soya for babies who can't tolerate a lactose-based milk. As I've mentioned, it is best to use with bespoke advice from a medical practitioner.

- **Other lactose-free milks**

Available over the counter and on prescription in the UK, lactose-free milks (as with soya formulas) use glucose as their main carbohydrate, which isn't so great for developing teeth. Lactose intolerance is rare and shouldn't be confused with cow's milk allergy. If these milks are used, it should be under medical supervision and for as short an amount of time as possible.

- **Extensively hydrolysed and amino acid milks**

Also known as 'hypoallergenic milk', these milks are available on prescription for mixed-fed and fully formula-fed babies diagnosed with cow's milk protein allergy (CMPA). Most babies respond well to an extensively hydrolysed milk where the milk protein is broken down. However, if the symptoms are very severe and the extensively hydrolysed milk isn't cutting it, an amino acid-based formula should be given instead.

- **Pre-term formulas**

If a premature baby is not having breast milk, they will be prescribed a specific formula designed for early arrivals. This will typically have more energy, protein and key micronutrients such as iron and vitamin D than a standard first milk formula.

Marketed from 6 months

- **Sleepy milks**

In the UK there is now only one brand specifically marketing a milk with cereal thickeners to help babies settle for bedtime. There is no evidence to support the claim that this helps and any milks with cereals added are not recommended. The carbohydrate content is very high and can lead to dental decay, especially if babies do not have their teeth brushed after drinking this milk. It's also very expensive.

- Follow-on milk

Follow-on milks were introduced by companies to enable them to advertise their brands whilst getting around the advertising laws that prevent them from marketing formula for babies under 6 months. It really is as simple as that. The World Health Organization and the UK's Department of Health agree that they are nutritionally unnecessary and that the only milk a formula-fed baby needs throughout the first 12 months is a standard first milk.

- Growing up/toddler milks

These milks are another way to instil insecurity in parents about their child's nutrition, and a ruse by the companies to make more cash. They are wholly unnecessary. They are very sweet, which can lead to some little ones getting hooked on the need for milk and sweetened foods. Despite having some extra nutrients such as iron and vitamin D, toddlers do not need this fortification in milk unless they have a very restricted diet.

From 12 months old, any full-fat pasteurised animal milk (cow, goat or sheep) is suitable. For toddlers who are on a cow's milk-free diet, there are unsweetened fortified toddler milks based on oats, soya, hemp or nuts available. These milks do tend to have less energy and nutritional content than animal milks (they may be missing out on iodine or riboflavin) so once again, go and chat to a paediatric nutritionist or dietician where you can. Any unmodified rice milk should be completely avoided for under 5s as it has a proportionally high level of arsenic.

DIY formula

There are countless blogs and vlogs about how to make home-made formula but is it really a good idea? Health authorities don't think so. The ingredients might not stack up to everything a baby needs and there is a considerable risk that the making and storage methods of homemade formula would fall short of those necessary to eliminate the risk of serious bacterial infections in a baby.

Preparing and storing formula

As with breast milk, prepping and storing formula milk safely is crucial to keeping a baby happy and healthy. Two areas to be particularly mindful of are:

- Even before you open the seal of the tin, powdered formula is not a sterile product and therefore making up the milk with hot water and preparing bottles as they're needed (and not in advance) is key to killing off and keeping any potential harmful bacteria at bay. Even in a fridge, bacteria can still multiply, albeit slowly. The two species of concern are salmonella and cronobacter sakazakii.
- Using the right amount of powder for a specific volume of water ensures that it is not too dilute (and therefore lower in calories and nutrients) or over-concentrated (which puts pressure on a baby's kidneys to handle the additional protein and electrolytes) possibly leading to dehydration, constipation and serious illness.

Always use fresh water from the cold tap to boil rather than from the hot tap. Hot water may have been stagnant in your storage tank for a while before using, so is not as fresh as the cold tap. Additionally, there is a small chance that if you have old plumbing the lead can leach into hot water. Try to avoid using water that has been re-boiled as it may potentially have levels of some minerals that are too high.

If you are using bottled water, remember that this isn't sterile and will still need to be boiled before use to kill off any bacteria in both the powder and the water itself. There is also some concern that bottled water could contain high levels of sodium or sulphates, though most bottles in the UK have sodium and sulphates well within recommended levels and even below the level of some regional tap water. To be on the safe side, always check that it has less than 200mg/l of sodium (Na) and 250mg/l of sulphate (SO4).

The water should be at least 70°C when the powder is added to it, so don't leave it for any longer than 30 minutes after boiling.

Once the water and the bottle equipment are ready to go, there are a few more steps before it is ready:

1. Wash your hands and any work surfaces thoroughly (using the inside of the steriliser lid is a clean, handy place to have the bottle equipment).
2. Measure out the required amount of water into the bottle.
3. Measure out the powder using the scoop provided and add to the water, being extra sure to level each scoop flat to avoid over-doing it.
4. Screw on the teat (try to avoid touching the tip of the teat) and then the bottle cap.
5. Give it a good shake until all the powder has dissolved.
6. Finish it off by swirling the bottle around in gentle circles to help knock out any excess bubbles.
7. If you need to give it straight away, run the bottle under a cold tap or put it in a container with cold water until it is warm but not hot, being careful to avoid getting the water on the top of the bottle.

Formula preparation machines

You may well have seen that there are machines now on sale that suggest they take the hassle out of making up formula. Whilst they do take away the time required to boil and cool the water, users still have to clean the bottles and measure the powder, whilst also taking time every now and then to maintain the machine. First Steps Nutrition Trust, a well-respected independent public health nutrition charity, suggests that both money and time can be saved by using vacuum flasks instead of one of these machines. To quote their work:

> If boiling water is kept in a full 500ml vacuum flask, the water will remain above 70°C for about 3 hours. A 1l vacuum flask filled with boiling water will still contain water at above 70°C for at least 6 hours, and offers a much simpler and cheaper solution for some families.

This hack is often used by families during the night to avoid having to leave the bedroom and attempt to stay awake over the boiling kettle.

Currently there is a scarcity of independent evidence that proves the machines are indeed safe and researchers remain unconvinced that the amount of hot water they use is enough to eliminate all the potential bacteria in the milk. Therefore medical bodies do not recommend them.

Storing made-up bottles of formula

Where it isn't possible to make up bottles on the go, the NHS recommends sticking within the following time limits for storing made-up formula:

- Room temperature: 2 hours
- Cool bag with ice pack: 4 hours
- Fridge: 24 hours

Should you then need to warm the bottle up you can either use an official bottle warmer or simply stand it in a jug or large mug of hot water. As with breast milk, never use a microwave as it may heat the milk unevenly.

We used to take a bottle of pre-mixed formula up to bed or when we were out and about but our daughter became fussy, refusing to drink anything but freshly mixed powder. While out and about, most places are happy to give hot water to warm the bottle. We found this easier than trying to make one up in advance and keep it warm or stop it spilling. We also bought a small plastic container that held 3 pre-measured portions of powdered formula, which was an absolute essential.

Chelsea

How much and how often to give a formula-feed

The amount of formula milk a baby will drink is not comparable to the amount of breast milk. While a good place to start for guidance is on the side of the tin, keep these points in mind:

- Babies (as for us) aren't built to have the same number of calories at strictly fixed times day in day out.
- At some feeds they will be hungrier than others. They will have some days when they are less bothered and then catch up on other days.
- They may want to suck on something even if they're not hungry. Breastfed babies not only suckle for nutrition but for comfort and they can change their pattern of doing this at the breast so that they aren't actively drinking. Bottle-fed babies can't do this without taking in both unwanted air and unnecessary additional calories. At times like this, a dummy can provide an alternative way of soothing them.
- Babies are all different sizes and their appetites will vary accordingly.
- Responsively feeding them according to their cues, using a technique known as 'paced bottle-feeding', outlined ahead, will help you to tell what is right for them.

With all this in mind, here is a *rough* guideline, to take with a pinch of salt, for how much and how often a formula-fed baby may feed in their first year. If your baby feeds more than or less than this and is happy and growing appropriately, they are having the right amount for them.

Age	Varying amounts per feed through the day/ night	Number of feeds in 24 hours
Birth–2 weeks	Increasing from 15–75ml (0.5–2.5oz)	7–8
2 weeks–2 months	75–105mls (2.5–3.5oz)	6–8
2–3 months	105–180mls (3.5–6oz)	5–7
3–6 months	120–210mls (4–7oz)	5–7
6–9 months	150–240mls (6–8oz) reducing as solid foods increase	4–5
9–12 months	105–210 mls (3.5–7oz)	3–4

Positioning for a bottle-feed

First up, bottle propping is never a great idea. That is any type of hands-free feeding, using a pillow, rolled up blanket or even some devices that can be bought specifically for this purpose, to support the bottle in a baby's mouth. There's no glossing over it – it's dangerous and should be avoided at all costs. It leaves the baby at the mercy of the flow of milk leading to a risk of choking, chest infections and over-feeding. On a less severe, but still important note, when a baby is given a bottle lying flat in their cot, it can trigger milk to travel inside their middle ear, potentially causing infant ear infections, and to also pool in their mouth, leading to dental decay. And since babies gain so much comfort and healthy brain development from having close human contact, with bottle propping they would be missing out on these opportunities.

So, is there a *right* way to give a bottle? As with breastfeeding, there are of course different ways to hold your baby on your body during a bottle-feed. They could be in your arms (skin-to-skin if you'd like), sitting close to your chest on your lap, sitting on your knees facing towards you and so on. If you have more than one baby to feed and they both need a bottle at the same time, the safest option (if you can't hold one or either in your arms) is to sit within reach in front of them whilst they are sitting in an upright baby bouncer, car seat or other supportive place (perhaps on a feeding pillow in your crossed legs). This way you can keep an eye on both babies and hold their bottles safely at the same time. When one baby needs to stop, then stop feeding both so that you can attend safely to both babies.

When a baby drinks a bottle quickly they are likely to end up more windy, over-fed and uncomfortable, compared to if things slowed down a bit. Think of a huge blowout meal and that tender feeling of needing to go and collapse afterwards! The speed of milk flow from a bottle is also a crucial factor in helping to minimise any potential problems for babies who are also breastfeeding. Where a baby gets used to a fast flow from the bottle, they may well start getting agitated on the breast when the same thing doesn't happen. Here are some useful principles to bear in mind, based on the method of paced bottle-feeding which allows her to control the feed as much as possible herself.

1. Hold her in an upright position where you can look at each other's face. When a baby is laid back they will not have any control of the flow and will be much more likely to gulp the milk down, possibly splutter and get a bit fretful. They will also have a tougher time indicating when they have had enough and could well drink more than they need. Being able to connect and see each other is a basic part of using this moment as both bonding and healthy brain-building time. If you

are holding her on one side of your body, aim to switch sides on alternate feeds (or whenever you remember), so that she experiences facing in both directions. This enhances her eye development and eye-hand coordination. It will help prevent both of you from getting a stiff neck and will also help you not to get one potentially sore arm and shoulder.

2.   **Allow the teat of the bottle to brush against her nose and upper lip.** This is a respectful way of calmly asking your baby if she's ready for her milk, so that she can reach up to the teat with an open mouth and take it if she'd like to. It's also an important reminder for breastfed babies that the nipple doesn't just land in her mouth and will help to support a good attachment at the breast.

3.   **As she 'asks' for the bottle with an open mouth, place the teat inside her mouth as deeply as possible.** By taking as much of the teat into her mouth as she can, she will be encouraged to sustain an open mouth to support her oral development as well as attachment back on the breast, if that's relevant for her.

4.   **Keep the bottle held in a horizontal position.** If there is milk in the part of the teat that is in her mouth, don't worry about seeing air outside her mouth. Holding the bottle in this way is helpful to allow her to be in control of the flow.

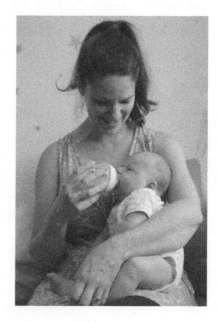

5.   **Give her lots of breaks.** Offer up to 2–3 every minute for babies in their first few months.

Gently bring the end of the bottle down towards the ground to stop the flow (it may stay in her mouth or come out completely). Hold it down for a few seconds and as she signals for more by starting to suck again or if she opens her mouth for the teat, put it back in using the same thing you did earlier in steps 2 and 3. Each gap in feeding need only be a few moments. This prevents the eyes-too-big-for-my-tummy guzzle and allows the feed to slightly resemble the suck-swallow-pause rhythm of breastfeeding, ensuring that she is able to have some regulation over her own appetite – a very important life lesson that starts right here.

6. **Enjoy it!** Feeding your baby provides cherished time together and yet, with the hustle and bustle of life, it is easy just to see it as one more thing on the to-do list. Wherever you are and whatever is going on around you, try and take a little time to give yourself an inward (or an outward!) smile and soak up this moment. Nikki has some brilliant quick pointers to help.

Nikki's Zen Zone

Peacefully surrender into the moment
During a bottle-feed you often get a chance to really see the whole of your child's precious face. Try spending a few moments really noticing all their tiny details – the miniscule hairs above their lip, the shape of their eyebrows, the curve of their ear lobes or the different colours in their eyes.

If you've arrived at this point and are bottle-feeding with any reluctance, it can help to remember some of these kind words whenever you're wavering about doing the right thing: *I make decisions which serve everyone's needs and I am in control of what to worry about.*

7.   Watch her signals when time's up or she needs a wind. Check back in Chapter 4 for recognising cues. When she is showing you that she's had enough, resist the urge to cajole her into finishing off the bottle. Having an empty bottle is not necessarily a sign of a successful feed; a happy and settled baby is what to aim for.

Bottle-feeding in this way should take around 10–20 minutes or longer. It's understandably tempting and sometimes unavoidable to hurry things along a bit when life is getting in the way. If that has to happen occasionally, don't worry or feel bad, just aim to stick with this as much as you can at other times.

Common bottle-feeding issues

The most common bottle-feeding problems that I see are babies who aren't very keen to suck, are gagging or are spilling lots of milk from the corners of their mouth.

For rectifying these issues there may be easy resolutions, such as:

- Changing the teat shape and/or flow
- Adjusting the position she is held in for the feed
- Doing some more winding
- Experimenting with warming or cooling the milk
- Watching her cues and figuring out whether she is hungry or if it's something else

Occasionally something more significant may be going on such as reflux, tongue-tie, low muscle tone or structural tension from pregnancy or birth. If you are at all concerned, talk to a health professional such as a midwife, health visitor, GP, lactation consultant or osteopath. You will be given further advice and a possible referral to a paediatrician or speech and language ther-apist if necessary.

See Chapter 4 for other concerns around crying, wind, colic, constipation and allergy.

Moving from a bottle to a cup

Dentists, dieticians, health visitors and pretty much anyone else who has anything professionally to do with babies, advise that they are introduced to a cup from around the age of 6 months and aim to ditch the bottle completely by 12–18 months. Learning to sip from a cup, rather than suck on a bottle, serves several purposes:

- It helps to ensure she is not drinking too much milk and missing out on being hungry for other food.
- It improves dental and ear health as less milk pools in her mouth.
- It improves development by building up muscles for chewing and talking.

The switch is quick and easy for some babies, while others will want to steadfastly stand their ground. The tips below are also relevant to introducing water or other milk (if you'd like to) to breastfed babies. Here are some ideas to have a crack at:

- Experiment with a few different cups if your first option isn't making headway. They should be free-flow (i.e. the liquid comes out if it is upside down) as cups with valves require a similar action from the baby as on a bottle.
- It's probably going to get messy, so start with water at mealtimes. Try to keep your happy game-face on, even if it gets flung around. Gently remind and demonstrate to her what to do with it. If she sees that flinging it on the floor elicits a sudden response from you (even if it's a shouty one), it'll only spur her on to do it again and see if she gets the same response. This isn't her

being tricky, she's just figuring out the basics of cause and effect.

- Give her tons of calm positive reinforcement when she does have a drink, for example, 'You are drinking so well, Daddy's very proud of you.'
- Once she is used to water in the cup, start offering some of her daytime bottle-feeds in a cup. Over time, slowly begin to water these down as she starts to take more and more solid foods. You will probably find that by doing this gradually, she will start to lose interest in the milk.
- Mix up the routine. For example, if she comes into your bed for a bottle in the morning, get straight out of bed and head to the kitchen or living room for a play and a snuggle somewhere different.
- When it comes to switching the bedtime bottle to a cup, try giving her some bottled milk first, then go to brush teeth, before coming back and offering some water in a cup whilst you have a cuddly story or song.

AFFIRMATIONS

- I enjoy feeding my baby
- It's OK to find this hard and I am handling it
- I am the right parent for my baby, just the way I am
- I feed my baby with love

7

Starting solids

Starting solid foods is an exciting milestone. My heart does flips watching their little faces grimace and light up as they start to explore this whole new world. Most parents care deeply about wanting 'to do the right thing' but what does that mean? In this chapter we will look at:

- When to get going with solids
- What babies need to eat to support optimal nutrition
- Our attitudes towards eating and why it's important when feeding babies
- How to start giving solids
- What kit is useful and what is not
- Keeping safe when preparing and giving foods
- What foods to give and what to avoid
- Suggested feeding routines

When to get going with solids

The official guidance in the UK is to start solid foods at around 6 months old. This is based on the optimal growth and readiness of breastfed babies, in addition to when they start to need additional nutrients to complement their milk. Policy-makers are in agreement that the guidance is still applicable, regardless of being breast or formula-fed.

On an individual basis, some parents do decide to start earlier than 6 months. These decisions can be based on common misinterpretations of the signs of readiness for solids, as we will review shortly. Whilst I fully advise following the guidance, this chapter does provide information to ensure that if you still choose to start earlier, that this might proceed as safely and as appropriately as possible.

In general, waiting until around the 6-month mark means:

- His digestive system is fully ready to start accepting food
- He will be ready and willing to chew as he will have lost the reflexive 'tongue thrust' (forwards and backwards movement) that younger babies have and be able to move his tongue in a more mature and complex way
- More breast milk for breastfed babies and thus a greater impact of all its benefits
- A lower chance (for all babies) of developing obesity later in life
- Possible protection against high blood pressure later on
- Less hassle for parents by not having to add in extra work earlier

The myths

Myths abound on what indicates when the timing's right, so let's clear up the main ones right here.

- **Waking up at night (or increased waking) means time for food. NOT true!**

Babies can start to wake more often around the 4–5-month mark due to a spurt in their development. However, extra milk feedings is what they really need and benefit from at this point.

- Giving 'first tastes' of purées from 4–6 months will prevent fussy feeding. NOT true!

This theory has never been supported by any evidence.

- Big babies or babies reaching a certain weight need food earlier. NOT true!

Being on one of the upper centiles of the growth chart has no bearing whatsoever on their digestive system being ready for food. Conversely, these babies benefit more from waiting and not being over-fed.

- Small babies need food earlier. NOT true!

As above, being of *any* weight does not reflect that their body is ready to healthily accept food. If there is a worry about slow weight gain this signals the need for a thorough assessment of breast and/ or bottle-feeding and ways to maximise milk intake if necessary. First foods are low in calorie content and will only displace the more calorific and nutritious milk.

- Chewing on fists indicates time for food. NOT true!

Babies use their highly sensitive mouths as a way to explore the world and will generally shove anything in there that they can get their hands on, including their fists themselves, to feel and experience it. If babies are feeling their teeth start to come through this is also likely to up the antics.

- The baby is hungry for more and more formula. NOT true!

As we have covered already, the ingredients in formula milk are set and therefore as a baby grows they will need more and more of it to meet their needs. This does not necessarily suggest that they are ready for solids.

- Breast milk is low on iron. NOT true!

On a like-for-like basis it does appear that breast milk has less iron than formula. However, this is intended by nature. Iron in breast milk is absorbed significantly more easily than iron in formula (around 50 per cent versus 2–9 per cent) and therefore it doesn't need to be as prolific to start with. Research has shown that *most* breastfed babies will have the right amounts of iron until at least 6 months, if not a little longer.

- **The baby is reaching for food. NOT true!**

Babies learn through mirroring the behaviour of others and if they see someone reaching for food they will likely try out the same. As with sucking on their fists, this doesn't reflect that their gut is ready to receive this food, simply that they are exploring smells and textures.

True signals that a baby is ready for solid food

These are:

- He can sit up with little or no support
- He has good head control
- He can pick up and bring food to his mouth in a controlled manner
- He is around 6 months old

Some great ways to involve your baby in mealtimes from around 4 months of age and teach him about food, *without* feeding him, can be:

- Carry him in a forward-facing sling or carrier whilst shopping for food and preparing meals
- Bring him with you to sit at the table on your lap or in a highchair
- Offer him baby-friendly bowls, plates, spoons and cups to play with
- Freeze EBM or formula in ice lolly moulds and then offer it to him as a lolly or as smashed up milky chips to play with and suck on

What about babies who were born prematurely?

There is currently little research that concludes precisely when there is a 'best' time to introduce foods to a premmie and, of course, it all depends on their individual situation. Generally you will want to look for the same signs as those given above, although some premature babies will take longer to sit on their own, for instance. Most professionals advise to start when you feel the time is right somewhere between their corrected age of 4–6 months (i.e. from the time that they were due, not the time of their birth).

Our baby was 5 months corrected (6.5 months actual age) when she started showing all the signs. We gave her some avocado to hold on to and she hoovered it up. It was really exciting to see her moving on after all she'd been through.

James

What babies need to eat to support optimal nutrition

You may hear the phrase 'food before 1 is just for fun', with the implication that it is purely about experiencing and getting used to different textures and flavours, rather than about any nutritional need. Whilst this is a crucial aspect of introducing food, and milk is still the most important part of their diet, there are some nutritional requirements (especially zinc and iron) that babies need from additional sources for optimal health and development. Perhaps the saying should be 'food before 1 is *mostly* for fun'.

The table below highlights the main nutrients that babies require and good sources, outside milk, to find them.

Nutrient	Why it's important	Good sources
Protein	Growth, maintaining and repairing body tissues and to make enzymes controlling many body functions	Meat, full-fat dairy, eggs, beans such as cannellini, kidney, black and adzuki, lentils, tofu, hummus, soya, ground nuts, nut butters, seeds, wholegrains, quinoa, oats
Carbohydrate	Complex carbohydrates provide essential energy for the nervous system, muscle and brain function and gut health (from fibre) Simple carbohydrates (including refined and processed foods such as biscuits, sweets, cakes, processed white bread and soft drinks) cause sharp spikes and falls in blood sugar and can negatively impact mood, memory, behaviour and gut health	Wholegrains, fruit, vegetables, pulses (e.g. lentils), oats, beans, sweet potato
Fats	Important source of energy and essential roles in immunity, nervous and circulatory system function and general health *Note: It's best to avoid/limit transfats, which are known to cause inflammation and poor health. These are found in deep-fried foods, fast-food and processed foods such as shop-bought cakes, pies and processed meat*	Unsaturated: olive oil, avocado, oily fish, chicken, eggs, nuts, seeds (such as linseed), edamame beans Saturated: fatty meats, full-fat dairy,* coconut oil *should be full-fat for under twos

Nutrient	Why it's important	Good sources
Iron	Having energy, fighting off infections, brain development *Absorption of iron is helped if eaten alongside vitamin C and hindered if eaten alongside dairy products*	Meat, fortified cereals and white flour, salmon, eggs, tuna, tofu, chickpeas, black-eyed peas, soya, lentils, beans (e.g. lima, kidney and haricot beans), seeds, dried fruit, dark green leafy vegetables, nut butters, quinoa
Calcium	Healthy bones and for the transmission of nerve signals, muscle movement and many other functions	Dairy, tofu, bony tinned fish, seeds, ground nuts, nut butters, broccoli, pak choi, okra, cabbage, figs, fortified foods and drinks (e.g. fortified plant-based milks and anything with fortified flour)
Vitamin A	Vision, growth, immune function and normal development of bodily tissues	Vegetables (particularly sweet potato, spinach, carrots and kale), fruits, red meat, oily fish, eggs, cheese
Vitamin B12	Works with folate and B6, essential for making red blood cells and a healthy nervous system	Meat (red, chicken and turkey), dairy, eggs, fortified cereals and plant-based milks
Vitamin C	Growth and repair of body tissues	Many fruits and vegetables, especially citrus fruit, berries, kiwi, tomatoes, spinach, cabbage, Brussels sprouts, pepper, kale and cauliflower

Nutrient	Why it's important	Good sources
Vitamin D	Helps calcium absorption and potentially has many roles in general health	Egg yolk, oily fish (e.g. salmon, mackerel, sardines, trout, fresh tuna), mushrooms, fortified cereals, margarine
Vitamin E	Strong antioxidant helping to protect the body from damage	Many fruits and vegetables, nuts (e.g. almonds, hazelnuts), vegetable oils and sunflower seeds
Vitamin K	Healthy blood clotting and keeps calcium levels balanced	Leafy green vegetables, meat, eggs, oily fish
Folate	Producing and looking after new cells	Green vegetables, lentils, fortified foods (e.g. pasta, cereals and bread), salmon, avocado
Zinc	Growth and general health	Kidney and soya beans, shellfish, meat, eggs, wholegrains, full-fat dairy, lentils, ground nuts, sesame seeds, tofu
Iodine	Needed to make thyroid hormones that are essential for growth, metabolism and brain development	Full-fat dairy, white fish, eggs

Reflecting on our attitudes towards eating and why this is important when feeding babies

Babies are born to be intuitive little eaters. And whilst they know what smells and feels good to them, it can take a while for the gagging to cease (more on this later). Some more cautious babies may need additional time to settle happily in a high chair and/or readily accept new tastes on a consistent basis. It is not unusual to find that babies need to see, smell, touch and taste a certain food on up to 10 or more different occasions before this happens.

Whilst this is going on, you will often find that a ton of your lovingly prepared food is either played with, straight-up rejected, ends up on the floor or smeared around just about everywhere. It can all sometimes feel like a punch in the stomach. Is it a reflection on our capability or success as individual parents or on the strength of the relationship we have with our babies? It isn't. It *really* isn't. This is all a completely normal and natural part of learning to explore and feel safe with food, coexisting alongside their cognitive stage of learning about movement along with cause and effect. For instance, babies of this age group are subconsciously working out the answers to questions such as, What does this broccoli do if I squidge it? If I let go of it, what will happen? Where will it go? How far will it travel? How will people react?, and so on.

When these feeding behaviours are experienced negatively by us, it is common and natural to build up feelings of annoyance, defensiveness, stress, anxiety, self-doubt and even fear. I've felt these moments (especially when my energy reserves have generally fallen off a cliff), when the hackles go up and I can feel everything tensing, my breathing changing and my voice simmering over into the red. As we know, babies are perceptive little souls and quickly recognise when we feel this way. Any increased anxiety we hold over choking, for instance, can lead to anxiety in the baby and rejection of food. Likewise, worrying about whether they are eating enough or doing 'the right thing' can inadvertently put pressure on babies to 'behave', making them eat more when they don't want it. This could potentially put them right off mealtimes and allow a cycle of negativity around food to kick off.

Before getting started, I believe that it's important to take some time to gently reflect on your own relationship with food and beliefs around eating behaviours, without criticism of yourself or others. For instance, were you brought up to 'be good' by finishing everything on your plate, told you couldn't have or do something until you've finished up first, or that you were naughty if you made a mess? This kind of unconscious conditioning could well influence and trigger uncomfortable feelings and attitudes in ourselves, when it comes to feeding our own children.

This may feel particularly pertinent to you if you have or have had an eating disorder, and you would not be on your own if you find that starting to give your baby solids is a particularly difficult time. If you do have any concerns, try not to hang back in talking about it with any professionals involved in your care as they will fully understand.

Ponder point

Taking a step back to see things more objectively can do wonders in lessening the impact of any stress, boosting your enjoyment of the whole process and thus helping your baby grow to love and have a positive relationship with eating themselves.

Note down any specific words that come to mind when considering your own thoughts and behaviours to do with food and eating in general.

Where do you believe these have come from?

Are they helping you as a parent now? If so, how? If not, in what way might they be unhelpful?

If you feel that you need to explore this further, write down who you would like to get in touch with to help support you, e.g. your GP, health visitor, therapist, family and friends.

It's hard when they seem to like something one week and not the next and I panicked a lot about what to introduce when and how quickly. Eventually I became so confused by all the information out there and just said, 'Sod it! Let's make it up as we go along!' Me relaxing helped her relax and things flowed much better after that. Even now, I don't panic when she rejects a food she's previously inhaled; we don't fancy the same food every day, so why should our babies?!

Chelsea

How to start giving solids

There are no hard and fast rules about following one exact method to the letter when starting to give solids and there are different routes to go down depending on the age of your baby and what your personal preference is.

The process of starting out is often referred to as complementary feeding since, for at least the first few months, any food given is *in addition* to a baby's milk rather than being in place of it. Accordingly, this term has officially replaced the old-school weaning terminology, which is interpreted by many to mean coming off the breast or other milk.

Spoon-feeding

If you are starting to give food before 6 months, and particularly if your baby is not showing the physical signs of readiness listed before, it is safest to give smooth foods using a spoon or, if you prefer, your own (clean!) finger. Families choosing this option will generally transition from purées to mashed, and then to minced and chopped foods over the course of a few months.

This method can be labour intensive on the prepping side, which works perfectly if it's something you enjoy but not so much fun otherwise. It is also very important to move through these stages swiftly to avoid getting to a point where your baby struggles with harder foods because they haven't developed the skills to chew. Using the window of opportunity between 6–9 months to introduce firmer textures has been shown to be key in helping babies not to resist these further down the line.

Baby-led weaning (BLW)

If you want to avoid purées and spoon-feeding altogether, BLW could be the way forward for you. This is when a baby is offered actual pieces of foods to pick up and eat as they choose and is a method that has been fast gaining in parental and professional popularity since the early 2000s.

Although there are limited studies on BLW, it is widely felt that this method helps develop self-feeding skills earlier and, on the whole, leads to less food fussiness and a greater enjoyment of food. This is because babies experience what 'real' food looks and feels like without any pressure. This could be particularly helpful for able babies who might have had a trickier time with feeding to date, due to reflux or prematurity for example, and perhaps need to regain a sense of safety, control and pleasure with food. On top of this, observational evidence shows that BLW can also help prevent a baby from being over-fed because they have more self-control over what they do and don't eat.

Common worries with BLW are whether a baby gets enough food to meet both nutritional and energy requirements as well as choking. I can clear up the latter easily. If the baby is:

- developmentally ready to accept finger foods
- can sit up straight
- the food is prepared safely
- the baby is in control of when it goes in their mouth

there is no evidence to date that BLW poses any additional risk of choking over and above spoon feeding.

In terms of meeting energy and nutritional requirements the jury is still in deliberation, particularly over the question of iron. I figure that this is where common sense should lead the way. We know that when mothers have good iron levels in pregnancy and when there has been delayed cord clamping at birth, a breastfed baby is well set up to have enough iron stores until at least 6 months, and some evidence suggests up until around 8 months. However, where this is not the case, it is possible that following a strict BLW approach (particularly if meat is off the cards) could lead to low iron levels in the growing baby. Likewise, if a baby is gaining weight slowly around the time of starting food, and particularly if they aren't that bothered about experimenting with and trying out food for themselves, a solely-focused BLW approach may not suit them either.

Mixing it up

Of course, there is a third way, the middle-man between both. Whilst the official NHS guidance doesn't go so far as to endorse rigidly sticking with a BLW approach, it does encourage using finger foods from 6 months.

> We began at 6.5 months with a mix of finger food and purée. Baby was super-keen to feed himself so we followed his lead. Be prepared for a mess! We pop him in the kitchen sink to swill him down straight after!
>
> Laura

> I started at 26 weeks with BLW. Solids saw the end of reflux problems for my eldest and was a real turning point for us. I felt a little sad when my daughter first had something other than my milk – happily emotional!
>
> Ellen

> I started just before 6 months. My son was a good eater and we never really struggled with him. I made some purées at first and then did a mix of finger foods and purées. The best piece of advice I was given was to not make an issue of food if my son didn't want to eat what was offered or maybe had a period where he didn't eat much. It will only make it worse! When they're hungry they'll eat.
>
> Helen

The takeaway from all this is that there isn't a single 'right' or 'wrong' way for all babies and your best approach is taking a route that feels most intuitive to you. Regardless of your preferred approach, there are some useful and relevant things for everyone to help encourage happy little eaters.

Tips to follow

- Remember that quantity is not the game here so begin with a relaxed, happy and not desperately hungry baby. Give a breastfeed or bottle first and then offer some food around 20 minutes later. This way he will have more patience to give new things a go and you can be sure he is still getting the most important food of all – his milk. After a while (this may be a few weeks or months depending on your baby), start to increase the time between milk and food a little so that his appetite helps to gradually build up more interest.

- Offer foods when you have time to allow things to go at a leisurely pace and try and resist the urge to hurry things along.

- Maintain lots of eye contact, chat and have fun with him, giving him plenty of praise and encouragement.

- Continue using the principles of responsive feeding by watching out for his cues and going with his signals. Trusting these cues allows him to learn healthy eating habits by being in tune with his own body. So don't worry about fixating on portion sizes – once a certain amount has hit the floor and been smeared in various places, it's hard to know exactly what's gone in and what hasn't anyway. You will know when he's had enough when he turns his head from you, pushes food away, shuts his mouth and/or generally becomes irritable or cries.

- As he grows and feeding becomes more efficient, a useful *rough* guideline to follow is being led by the size of his palm for each food he has. For example, one meal may contain a portion of risotto the size of one palm, plus one or two palms of veggies, and then a palm-size yoghurt and piece of fruit. It's always better to start with a small amount, allow him to finish it up as he wants and then offer a little more if necessary, rather than overwhelming you both with a bigger portion to begin with.

- Resist forcing or pressurising him to eat anything that he isn't ready for or doesn't want. Any kind of coercion such as, 'We're not getting out of the highchair until this is finished' or 'I've made lots of effort so let's eat it up and make me happy', or putting food in a baby's mouth when they're not willing to accept it, will not only likely put him off mealtimes but is also a big choking risk.

- Keep things familiar and consistent as much as possible, e.g. sitting your baby in the same place at roughly similar times of day.

- If you are using spoons, give him his own spoon to hold as well. Let him dip the spoon in the food, touch it with his hands and hold the spoon you are holding (if he reaches for it) as you guide it towards his mouth. If you hold his hands away he is likely to become frustrated and the meal could start turning into a battle for control.

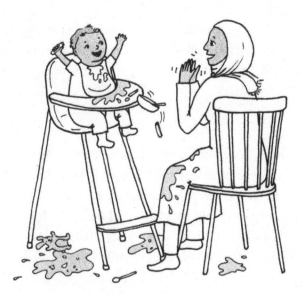

- Try to anticipate and accept that it can get messy. Mess is a great reflection of self-exploration. It is a short-term hit for helping him feel positive about food and learning to self-feed more quickly (and with less mess) in the longer-term. So whilst it might sometimes seem that there's more food 'out' than 'in', know that a happy baby is a big win.
- Model eating behaviour for him. Try and eat something, even if it's something small, whilst you are feeding him. The more he sees you eating and enjoying it, the more he'll want to try it out for himself.
- Introduce a wide variety of foods over the first few months to encourage acceptance and interest. There is no need to wait a few days between offering each new food as was once thought. The only time when this is useful is when starting with any of the common allergenic foods so you can watch out for any possible signs of reaction.

Gathering the Kit

'Stuff overload' doesn't abate when it comes to starting solid foods. Here's my rundown, drawing on my own experience and that of many of my clients, for what's hot and what's not.

Hot

- **Highchair.** Your choice will largely depend on your style, budget and availability of space. Whichever one you go for make sure that it is easy to clean. Padded, material-based highchairs do tend to be the hardest to clean and could drive you nuts. An alternative to a typical highchair is one that clips or screws directly on to your table.

- **Bibs.** If it's not the right time of year to strip off your baby and save all their clothes from obliteration, a long-sleeved bib is the next best option. Choose ones that are wipeable (e.g. neoprene or silicone) so you don't have to machine-wash them all the time.
- **Plates, bowls and cutlery.** If using plastic, make sure that it is in good condition and replace them when they become scratched to stop any potential leaching into food, particularly when washed at hot temperatures. If you want to save on plastic, go for stainless steel or wooden options.
- **Microwave steamer.** If you have a microwave, using a steamer is a cheap, easy and quick way to cook vegetables and fish.
- **Splash mat.** This goes under the highchair to protect your floor and make cleaning easier. Alternatively, you could use newspaper or bin liners.
- **Snack pots** for on the go. Ones that have lids designed for little hands to reach inside without spilling the snacks everywhere are brilliant.
- **Tupperware** or other storage boxes for freezing and keeping leftovers in the fridge.
- **Insulated picnic bag** for eating out.
- **Cups** (see page 244).

If you are making purées these two products can make life easier:

- **Silicone weaning cube trays** for the freezer
- **Food blender**

Not so hot

- **Netted bags** marketed to be a 'safe' way to feed babies. These do not allow a baby to learn to chew on their food, experience the texture or allow visibility of foods. They simply have to suck the food through the net.

- **Bowls and plates with suction caps** that (supposedly) stick on to the tray or table. These have mixed reviews and do often end up with food being slung across the room at greater force when the suction is broken.
- **Training cups with valves** inside the teat. A baby must suck on these in a similar way to a bottle, which unnecessarily delays giving them the opportunity to learn to control the flow of fluid themselves.

Keeping safe

Important health and safety tips:

- Always wash your hands and surfaces before preparing the food
- Keep any animals away from your food prepping area
- Wash all fruits and vegetables
- If you are storing the food, freeze it as soon as it is cooled (and mark it with the date)
- Defrost thoroughly and heat until it's steaming from the middle when it's time to use
- Never re-freeze any foods and throw away any reheated leftovers
- British Lion-marked eggs can be eaten runny* although this cannot be said for certain with other eggs
- Cook all shellfish thoroughly before giving to your baby
- Always keep your attention with your baby throughout their mealtime and ensure that they are in secure straps
- Ensure your baby is sitting up and not in a reclined position whilst they are eating

---

* Advice as per the Food Standard Agency (2017).

Gagging versus choking

An effortless way to keep a cool head around starting foods is to have a clear understanding of the difference between gagging and choking.

Almost all babies will gag on occasion (and sometimes frequently) when they first start solids. It is neither dangerous nor an indication that they don't like their food. Gagging is simply the body's natural defence against actual choking and a baby's gag reflex is much more pronounced than in an adult. If they can't deal with a piece of food, the gag reflex will be stimulated to help them move it towards the front of their mouth, where they will either spit it out or continue to chew on it. When this happens they will likely become flushed in the face and may splutter and cough. These are healthy signs that they're working the food out and the key thing for a parent or carer is to try and stay cool about it. If we look or sound worried or make sudden movements to 'help' they will think there's a problem and become worried too. Ironically this could possibly lead to an actual choking episode. The more a baby experiences gagging in a relaxed environment, the quicker they will figure out what to do with their food and the gagging episodes will decrease and eventually stop.

Choking is completely different and occurs when a piece of food has gone beyond the gag reflex and is blocking, or partially blocking, the airway. This is far less common and is largely preventable. A baby who is choking will go pale or slightly blue and be very quiet. If this ever happens, follow the basic first aid technique which involves back slaps over your lap and possible chest thrusts. Consider taking a first aid course that covers how to do this safely and appropriately. If you can't access one, have a look at online educational videos and make sure that everyone else taking care of your baby is aware of what to do as well.

Key points for minimising any choking episodes:
- Avoid all the classically hazardous foods listed in the following table.
- Always halve grapes, baby tomatoes and other similar-sized foods for under 5s

- Sit them fully upright for every meal. Babies should not be fed reclined in a bouncy chair or their buggy.
- Never catch them unawares by putting a spoon of food in their mouth without them having seen and acknowledged it first.
- Never put any finger foods in their mouth for them. Offer pieces on a tray or in your open palm so that they can take them and be in total control.
- Only ever give food when you can always see and easily reach them. Remember that choking is silent, so never give food whilst they are in the back of the car or whilst pushing them in a forward-facing buggy, for instance.

My daughter was about 18 months old nibbling on a piece of cheese when I had my back to her in the kitchen. I turned around and she was choking, for the first time ever. Eating cheese was something she did every day so I thought she could manage it fine.

Natalie

What foods to give and what to avoid

We'll get the what-not-to-gives out of the way to make way for all the yummy stuff coming up.

WHAT NOT TO GIVE Under 6 months	Under 1 year	Under 5 years
Gluten (e.g. bread, pasta, flour and oats) Allergenic foods (e.g. eggs, seeds, soya, nuts, fish and shellfish)	Honey (rarely it may contain a bacteria leading to infant botulism) Added salt and sugar Salty packaged foods Low-fat or diet foods	Whole grapes Whole baby tomatoes Hard sweets

WHAT NOT TO GIVE Under 6 months	Under 1 year	Under 5 years
Dairy (e.g. cheese, custard and yoghurt) Acidic fruits (e.g. berries)	Too much high-fibre foods (wholegrain bread and cereals as this will fill him up quickly) Strong spices, such as hot chilli powder or paprika Cow's milk or plant-based milks as a main drink (see box overleaf) Fruit juices, squash	Popcorn (that may have un-popped hard corn inside) Mini chocolate eggs Sticky toffee Marshmallows Whole nuts Sausage skin Chunks of hard fruit or vegetables Tea and coffee Fizzy drinks

WHAT TO GIVE If starting under 6 months	From 6 months
Vegetables Fruits Gluten-free cereal*	Pretty much anything and everything that is not listed in the 'what to avoid' table! Multi-vitamin with vitamins A, C and D†

---

* This could include shop-bought baby rice. Whilst baby rice has been a traditional staple for feeding babies for many years, it is now widely thought best to either avoid it completely or to give on an occasional basis if at all. It is not a necessary part of a baby's diet. Baby rice is a bland and highly-processed food that quickly converts to glucose when eaten. The fortified nutrients added to it (to replace those stripped by the processing) are not as easily absorbed as those from breast milk or fresh foods. Rice also contains a proportionally high amount of arsenic (a chemical found in the natural environment all around us) which has been linked to various cancers. As babies are tiny, giving baby rice on a frequent basis could mean that they inadvertently receive levels of arsenic higher than we'd wish.

† Current UK advice is for all babies to have a multi-vitamin from 6 months to 5 years (unless they are having more than 500mls of formula per day). Some brands contain more unnecessary additives and preservatives than others, so check the label if it bothers you.

Cow's milk and plant-based milk

Cow's milk is nutritionally very different from the formula made from it, with cow's milk containing higher protein and mineral levels and lower vitamin C and iron, compared with formula. It is also hard for babies to digest. Drinking it as a main drink under 1 can lead to nutritional deficiencies, digestive problems and dehydration. Again, for reasons of nutritional deficiency, plant-based milks aren't recommended as whole drinks either until at least babies are 1 year old, after which fortified versions are preferred. Whilst they can all be used in cooking (e.g. mashed potato, white sauces etc.), it is best to keep intake low.

Allergenic foods

Food allergies are thought to affect around 3–6 per cent of babies in developed countries, with the chances being higher for babies with parents or siblings who have an allergic condition such as asthma, eczema, hay fever, atopic dermatitis or food allergies. There is currently no indication that premature babies will develop food allergies any more than term babies.

The pendulum has swung back and forth in regards to when to first introduce these foods, although the general scientific consensus is now to go for it between 6–9 months old and aim not to delay them beyond 10–11 months (there is adequate evidence that doing so afterwards increases the chance of developing food allergies). There is no strong evidence that suggests starting before 6 months has any benefits for preventing allergy development (this goes for gluten and peanut as well, for which there has been much debate in the last 10 years). If there are allergies in your baby's immediate family, or if they have already been diagnosed with eczema or a food allergy, have a chat with your GP, health visitor or other health professional for one-to-one advice.

As and when you do introduce allergenic foods, start with small amounts such as a smear on your finger or a small spoonful and watch out for any reactions, both immediately and across the next few days. If your baby has any of the following call 999 without hesitation as these signs can indicate a rare anaphylactic reaction:

- Swollen tongue
- Sudden, persistent cough
- Hoarse cry and/or noisy breathing
- Difficulty breathing
- Pale, floppy, unresponsive

Less severe reactions may include swollen lips, face or eyes, an itchy rash, tummy pain, vomiting, diarrhoea, constipation, eczema and a runny or blocked nose.

Make a note of anything you see and hold off giving the suspected food again for at least another week or two (if anaphylaxis was not involved) until any symptoms have fully settled down. This way you will have a clearer picture whether you see another reaction the next time this food is given. If you have any worries at all chat to your GP, health visitor or other health professional. They may then advise you to follow a specific elimination diet or refer you on for specific advice to ensure that your baby will still be receiving the nutrients they need. They'll advise you when and how it may be safe and appropriate to reintroduce the food, to work towards developing tolerance. You may also be referred to a specialist allergy clinic if there are significant concerns such as anaphylaxis, faltering growth, severe reflux and/or eczema. The likelihood of if, and when, a baby will develop tolerance to a troublesome food or food group largely comes down to how severe the reaction is and what the food or food group is.

If you don't see any reaction when introducing new foods, it helps to carry on offering them regularly to keep their body tolerating them.

Vegetarian and vegan diets

It is feasible to ensure that a baby has all they need from a purely plant-based diet, although it takes some extra consideration and organisation.

The nutrients to keep a particular eye on are protein, fats, iron, iodine, calcium, zinc and vitamin B12. Aim for 1–2 daily servings of these nutrients (in addition to breast milk or formula) from around 8–9 months onwards as milk intake slowly starts to decrease. Without dairy products, the minerals listed here are confined to specific sources, and it is particularly hard to get iodine and vitamin B12 from suitable sources for babies. Speak to a paediatric dietician for advice on supplementation and meal ideas if you are raising your baby on a vegan diet.

Commercial baby foods

Pouches and jars of baby food are everywhere we look and sell themselves as being a healthy and convenient option. As with everything we're sold, go forth with an open mind. Some brands are far superior in their nutritional content and flavours than others, so look beyond the fancy marketing and check out the ingredients. Often what is advertised as a main ingredient barely makes it into double per cent figures of the overall content. The caveat is that whilst convenient, packaged foods are very often expensive, sweet, too smooth for the baby's age, bland and less nutritious. They are certainly a useful fallback for busy times (I've been there, done it and am sure I will do so again!) but try and steer away from them becoming an everyday staple.

Serving it all up

- **4–6 months**

If you choose to start before 6 months (see page 246), use a blender or sieve to purée the food to make it smooth. Go with his flow in terms of the amount to give. This is likely going to be a few small spoons at each 'meal' to start with and gradually building up to 5, 10 and so on. Aim to be veggie-led first off, beginning with a single ingredient at a time such as carrot, broccoli, butternut squash, courgette, parsnip or sweet potato, before starting to combine them. There are no rules about when to do this apart from to remember that babies love taste and variety, so there is no reason not to mix things up when you feel the time is right. You could also add breast milk or formula if you wish, and potato is a useful thickener. Once he has had a variety of different savoury flavours then start to add fruits as well. Doing things the other way around *could* mean accepting veggies is a little trickier.

- **6–7 months**

As per the guidance, this is the ideal time to get started. Let things get interesting with textures and there is no reason to hold back from introducing iron-rich meat and other foods straight away. Water can start to be given at mealtimes. As long as this is from a clean water source this does not need to be boiled.

If you are spoon-feeding, you can either skip purées altogether and move straight to mashed foods or move through the purées stage in just a few days or weeks.

Ensure finger foods are cut to be around the width and length of an adult finger, so they are easy to pick up with the whole hand. For example, fingers of steamed carrot, courgette, pepper, sweet potato, banana, avocado, broccoli florets, chicken breast or lamb, stir-fried tofu, cheese, flaky fish, breadsticks and toast. Check that they are soft enough to be mashed in a mouth with no (or few) teeth and remove anything tricky to cope with such as skins, stringy or fatty bits. Also be sure to remove any stones, seeds or pips.

• **7–9 months**

As the amount of food being eaten gradually increases, begin to think about including something rich in iron, something energy-dense (such as potato, pasta, egg, beans, nut butter, banana, avocado or rice) and a vitamin-rich food source at each main meal. If you have a little toast fan, a simple, nutritious hack is to spread any of the following on toast fingers: hummus, fruit purée, nut butters, yoghurt, bean dip, avocado, chia seed jam, vegetable sauces – you name it.

Food life can also start getting fun by offering up more substantial dishes such as Bolognese, stews, thick soup, risottos, frittatas, savoury pancakes, quiche, muffin pizzas, fish cakes and pies. Don't be shy with using herbs, garlic and mild spices such as cinnamon for jazzing up flavours. The meals can either be mashed up, lumpy or simply as they come, although do break up any chunks of meat, fish and veg that could be a choking risk. This will also be the period to start lengthening the time between having milk and offering foods so that he gradually becomes more interested.

• **9–12 months**

By now, he is likely to be mastering a neat little pincer grip with his thumb and forefinger and may like to start playing about with picking up smaller foods such as peas and raisins. If you do give him raisins, ensure that they are not clumped together and, as with all finger foods, never put them in his mouth for him. He can also start to have firmer foods such as thicker wedges of hard cheese, raw carrot batons, strips of dried fruits, crackers and sugar-free flapjacks.

Babies of this age love to be the boss of their own cutlery. Offering foods that are easy to dig into that will cling to spoons and forks, such as mashed potato, polenta, risotto and thick (home-made) sauces, will greatly increase their confidence and skills.

Around this stage, the frequency of milk feeds tends to start decreasing as their appetite increases for solid foods. Occasionally babies might go right off their milk. Despite it still being a very important part of their nutrition, don't panic if it's being refused. It may be a case of them simply not being hungry for it, in which case slightly mixing up your routine or offering a little less food might sort things out. However, if he's really shut up shop then simply be mindful of adding in more milk (or dairy alternatives) into cooking, such as mashed potato, porridge, homemade custard, pancakes, scrambled egg and French toast, and offering yoghurts and cheese. Also look out for other foods rich in unsaturated fats, protein and calcium so you are confident he is receiving the nutrients he needs.

On the other end of the scale, you may be finding that he only wants milk and isn't bothered about food. This may be happening if he is filling up on lots of milk in the night, is still having milk feeds immediately before being offered foods and/or feels safer with the familiarity and security of milk rather than food. There are lots of tips on pages 260–62 to handle these situations and again, if in doubt, always chat to an understanding peer counsellor or professional.

Suggested routines

When introducing any routines, the principles of being guided by your baby's cues for when he wants and needs to breastfeed and/or bottle-feed still apply. This table provides a rough outline for bringing in mealtimes, if you want to give it a go, for you to flesh out with whatever additional milk feeds are necessary.

	4–6 months	6–7 months	7–9 months	9–12 months
Morning wake-up	Milk	Milk	Milk	Milk

Breakfast			Cereal, porridge, egg, toast, fruit, sugar-free pancake or yoghurt	As for 7–9 months
			Water	
Mid-morning	Milk	Milk	Milk	Milk and/or savoury snack
Lunch	Milk	Predominantly savoury meal (1 or 2 foods) Water	Predominantly savoury meal and pudding Water	Predominantly savoury meal and pudding Water
Mid-afternoon	Milk	Milk	Milk	Milk and/or savoury snack
Tea-time	Milk	Milk	Milk and/or savoury meal Water	Savoury meal and naturally-sweet pudding Water
Bedtime	Milk	Milk	Milk	Milk
During the night	Continue to have milk if waking and needing some. See Chapter 4 if you are worried about how often he may be waking and feeding.			

What to do if it's not going well

It's a fact of life that almost every baby will refuse to eat our food at some stage and it's human nature to feel an emotional response as a result. Checking in with ourselves at times like this, as Nikki suggests here, is one of the most important things we can do.

Nikki's Zen Zone

Shifting our minds into the positive

Our minds are like Velcro for negative experiences and Teflon for positive ones. This quirk of the human psyche is called the negativity bias and although it's seemingly unhelpful, it is the default setting of our minds.

Just knowing this can help us to realise when we may have been unjustifiably fixated on what isn't going well in our parenting journey, when there's almost certainly a lot of things which *are* working well – we've just forgotten to think about them.

Gratitude is one of the best easy tools we can use for shifting our perspective into the positive. In fact, over the past two decades studies have consistently shown that people who practise gratitude report fewer symptoms of illness, are happier and more optimistic.

The practise of gratitude is simple. You spend a few minutes recalling memories of things which have made you feel good within the last day. It works best when you think of small things such as the sunshine at the window, the softness of your bed and the closeness of a cuddle.

You can count these on your fingers or write them in a journal. I like to try for ten experiences but as few as three is enough to shift your mood. It's also a really nice one to do during feeding sessions or with older kids, counting on each finger little things which have brought us moments of joy.

If you feel that it is becoming an increasing issue, taking stock on the following points could help uncover why:

- Does he look worried or tense about eating?
- Is he ready to take more control and experiment with feeding himself?

- Is he feeling ill or teething?
- Is he too tired at mealtimes?
- Is the food at a temperature he enjoys?
- Is he hungry or has he filled up on milk and/or snacks?
- Are his portion sizes realistic?

Feeding issues can occasionally run deeper and, despite addressing all these things, he may be gaining weight very slowly or possibly even losing weight. If this happens, your GP should arrange for a referral to a paediatric dietician who may suggest a specific meal plan as well as fortifying his diet with specific energy-dense foods. If there are any additional worries, such as signs of an underlying disorder or unexplained weight loss, he should be referred as quickly as possible to see an appropriate paediatric specialist.

AFFIRMATIONS

- *I step back and see things from my baby's point of view*
- *I follow my intuition*
- *We have fun together during mealtimes*
- *When my baby does not eat, I know that this is not a reflection on my ability as a parent or on our relationship with each other*

Final thoughts

And so there it is – feeding a young baby in all its defining, messy, achingly beautiful and enduringly challenging glory. Feeding is not a cloneable one-way street. It is a distinctive, physical and emotional dance between you and your baby that can twist and turn and never be entirely predictable.

It's knowing that the is-it-just-me? moments are universal. It's knowing that whatever you feel is acceptable and valid. It's knowing that being informed and believing in yourself can influence the course of your feeding goals and help you ride the waves that can wash in with the tide. It's knowing that if plans shift about, there's never any blame or shame to lay at your feet. It's knowing that millions of parents and professionals all around the world get it and have your back.

We all have our own feeding stories. Each one filled with a different beginning, middle and end. But each one filled with love and ultimately playing out because we all do what we can to respond to our babies and to our own needs, in the best way we know how and with whatever resources we have in that time.

You are and will be enough. Reach out for help if you need it, listen to your heart and you will be dancing this feeding tango like you never knew you could bust moves before!

References

CHAPTER 1

Ballard O and Morrow AL (2013) Human milk composition: nutrients and bioactive factors. *Pediatr Clin North Am.* 60(1): 49–74.

Galante L, Milan AM, Reynolds CM, Cameron-Smith D, Vickers MH and Pundir S (2018) Sex-Specific Human Milk Composition: The Role of Infant Sex in Determining Early Life Nutrition. *Nutrients.* 10(9): 1194.

Lehmann GM, LaKind JS, Davis MH, Hines EP, Marchitti SA, Alcala C and Lorber M (2018) Environmental Chemicals in Breast Milk and Formula: Exposure and Risk Assessment Implications. *Environmental Health Perspectives.* 126(9).

Minchin M (2015) *Milk Matters: Infant Feeding & Immune Disorder.* BookPOD.

Renfrew MJ, Fox-Rushby J, Subhash P, Dodds R, Quigley M, Duffy S, McCormick F, Trueman P, Williams A (2012) Preventing disease and saving resources: The potential contribution of increasing breastfeeding rates in the UK, UNICEF UK. Baby Friendly Initiative. https://www.unicef.org.uk/babyfriendly/wp-content/uploads/sites/2/2012/11/Preventing_disease_saving_resources_policy_doc.pdf.

Tham R, Bowatte G, Dharmage SC, Tan DJ, Lau MX, Dai X, Allen KJ and Lodge CJ (2015) Breastfeeding and the risk of dental caries: a systematic review and meta-analysis. *Acta Paediatrica.* 104(467): 62–84.

https://placentarisks.org/hormones/.

Barrera C, Valenzuela R, Chamorro R, Bascunan K, Sandoval J, Sabag N, Valenzuela F, Valencia MP, Puigrredon C and Valenzuela A (2018) The Impact of Maternal Diet during Pregnancy and Lactation on the Fatty Acid Composition of Erythrocytes and Breast Milk of Chilean Women. *Nutrients.* 10(7): 839.

Salari P and Abdollahi M (2014) The influence of pregnancy and lactation on maternal bone health: A systematic review. *Journal of Family and Reproductive Health.* 8(4): 135–48.

Fernandez-Ruiz J, Gomez M, Hernandez M, de Miguel R and Ramos JA (2004) Cannabinoids and gene expression during brain development. *Neurotoxicity Research.* 6: 389–401.

Astley SJ and Little RE (1990) Maternal marijuana use during lactation and infant development at one year. *Neurotoxicology Teratology.* 12: 161–8.

http://www.hse.gov.uk/mothers/faqs.htm.

Doherty AM, Lodge CJ, Dharmage SC, Dai X, Bode L and Lowe AJ (2018) Human Milk Oligosaccharides and Associations with Immune-Mediated Disease and Infection in Childhood: A Systematic Review. *Frontiers in Pediatrics.* 6: 91.

Kramer MS and Kakuma R (2012) Optimal duration of exclusive breastfeeding. Cochrane Systematic Review. https://www.cochranelibrary.com/cdsr/doi/10.1002/14651858.CD003517.pub2/full.

Yan J, Liu L, Zhu Y, Huang G and Wang PP (2014) The association between breastfeeding and childhood obesity: a meta-analysis. *BMC Public Health.* 12: 1267.

Aune D, Norat T, Romundstad P and Vatten LJ (2014) Breastfeeding and the maternal risk of type 2 diabetes: a systematic review and dose-response meta-analysis of cohort studies. *Nutrition, Metabolism & Cardiovascular Diseases.* 24(2): 107–15.

Victoria CG, Bahl R, Barros AJD, Franca GVA, Horton S, Krasevec J, Murch S, Sankar MJ, Walker N and Rollins NC (2016) Breastfeeding in the 21st century: epidemiology, mechanisms, and lifelong effect. *The Lancet.* 387(10017): 475–90.

Chowdhury R, Sinha B, Sankar MJ, Taneja S, Bhandari N, Rollins N, Bahl R and Martines J (2015) Breastfeeding and maternal health outcomes: a systematic review and meta-analysis. *Acta Paediatrica.* 104(467): 96–113.

Luan NN, Wu QJ, Gong TT, Vogtmann E, Wang YL and Lin B (2013) Breastfeeding and ovarian cancer risk: a meta-analysis of epidemiological studies. *American Journal of Clinical Nutrition.* 98(4): 1020–31.

Dias CC and Figueiredo B (2015) Breastfeeding and Depression: a systematic review of the literature. *Journal of Affective Disorders.* 171: 142–54.

Winder K (2016) What's in Breast milk and What's in Formula? https://www.bellybelly.com.au/baby/ingredients-in-breast-milk-and-formula/.

WHO & UNICEF (2003) *Global Strategy for infant and young child feeding.* Geneva. https://www.who.int/nutrition/publications/infantfeeding/9241562218/en/.

Andreas NJ, Kampmann B and Le-Doare M (2015) Human breast milk: A review on its composition and bioactivity. *Early Human Development.* 91(11): 629–635.

Gao Z, Wang R, Qin ZX, Dong A and Liu CB (2018) Protective effect of breastfeeding against childhood leukemia in Zhejiang Province, PR China: a retrospective case-control study. *Libyan Journal of Medicine.* 13(1): 1508273.

Amitay EL and Keinan-Boker L (2015) Breastfeeding and Childhood Leukemia Incidence: a meta-analysis and systematic review. *JAMA Pediatrics.* 169(6).

Brown A (2017) Breastfeeding as a public health responsibility: A review of the evidence. *Journal of Human Nutrition and Dietetics.* 30(6): 759–70.

UNICEF (2017) Removing the barriers to breastfeeding: a call to action. https://www.unicef.org.uk/babyfriendly/wp-content/uploads/sites/2/2017/07/Barriers-to-Breastfeeding-Briefing-The-Baby-Friendly-Initiative.pdf. Accessed June 2019.

CHAPTER 2

Woody CA, Ferrari AJ, Siskind DJ, Whiteford HA and Harris MG (2017) A systematic review and meta-regression of the prevalence and incidence of perinatal depression. *Journal of Affective Disorders.* 219: 86–92.

Paulson JF and Bazemore SD (2010) Prenatal and postpartum depression in fathers and its association with maternal depression: a meta-analysis. *Journal of the American Medical Association.* 303(19): 1961–69.

Beck CT and Watson S (2008) Impact of Birth Trauma on Breastfeeding. *Nursing Research.* 57(4): 228–36.

Sacks A (2019) Matrescence: The Developmental Transition to Motherhood. https://www.psychologytoday.com/gb/blog/motherhood-unfiltered/201904/matrescence-the-developmental-transition-motherhood.

Machin A (2018) *The Life of Dad: The Making of a Modern Father.* Simon & Schuster UK.

Moberg KU (2014) *Oxytocin: The Biological Guide to Motherhood.* Praeclarus Press.

Kendall-Tackett K (2017) *Depression in New Mothers: Causes, Consequences and Treatment Alternatives* (3rd edn). Routledge.

CHAPTER 3

Center on the Developing Child (2007) *The Science of Early Childhood Development.* www.developingchild.harvard.edu/library.

Tsujimoto S (2008) The Prefrontal Cortex: Functional Neural Development During Early Childhood. *Neuroscientist.* 14(4): 345–58.

Sohn M, Youngmee A and Lee Sangmi (2011) Assessment of Primitive Reflexes in High-risk Newborns. *Journal of Clinical Medicine Research.* 3(6): 285–90.

Widstrom AM, Lija G, Aaltomaa-Michalias P, Dahllof A, Lintula M and Nissen E (2011) Newborn behaviour to locate the breast when skin-to-skin: a possible method for enabling early self-regulation. *Acta Paediatrica.* 100(1).

Mekonnen A, Yehualashet S, Bayleyegn D (2019) The effects of kangaroo mother care on the time to breastfeeding initiation among preterm and low birthweight infants: a meta-analysis of published studies. *International Breastfeeding Journal.* 14(12).

De Weerth C and Buitelaar JK (2007) Childbirth complications affect young infants' behaviour. *European Child & Adolescent Psychiatry.* 16(6): 379–88.

CHAPTER 4

https://www.unicef.org.uk/babyfriendly/wp-content/uploads/sites/2/2016/07/Co-sleeping-and-SIDS-A-Guide-for-Health-Professionals.pdf.

Li DK, Willinger M, Petitti DB, Odouli R, Liu L and Hoffman HJ (2006) Use of a dummy (pacifier) during sleep and risk of sudden infant death syndrome (SIDS): population based case-control study. *BMJ.* 332(7532): 18–22.

Moon RY, Tanabe KO, Yang DC, Young HA and Huack FR (2012) Pacifier Use and

SIDS. Evidence for a Consistently Reduced Risk. *Journal of Maternal and Child Health.* 16(3): 609–14.

Moore T and Ucko LE (1957) Night Waking in Early Infancy. *Archives of Disease in Childhood.* 32(164): 333–42.

Brown A and Harries V (2015) Infant Sleep and Night Feeding Patterns During Later Infancy: Association with Breastfeeding Frequency, Daytime Complementary Food Intake and Infant Weight. *Breastfeeding Medicine.* 10(5): 246–52.

Moon RY (2016) SIDS and Other Sleep-related Infant Deaths: Evidence Base for 2016 Updated Recommendations for a Safe Sleeping Environment. *Pediatrics.* 138.

Ball H (2003) Breastfeeding, Bed-Sharing and Infant Sleep. *Birth.* 30(3): 181–88.

Wiessinger D, West D, Smith L and Pitman T (2014) *Sweet Sleep: Nighttime and Naptime Strategies for the Breastfeeding Family.* Pinter & Martin Ltd.

Feldman R (2015) Mutual influences between child emotion regulation and parent-child reciprocity support development across the first 10 years of life: Implications for developmental psychopathology. *Development and Psychopathology.* 27: 1007–23.

Hookway L (2019) *Holistic Sleep Coaching: Gentle Alternatives to Sleep Training for Health and Childcare Professionals.* Praeclarus Press.

Doan T, Gay CL, Kennedy HP, Newman J and Lee KA (2014) Nighttime breastfeeding behavior is associated with more nocturnal sleep among first-time mothers at one month postpartum. *Journal of Clinical Sleep Medicine.* 10(3): 313–19.

Chapter 5

Boundy EO, Dastjerdi R, Spiegelman D, Fawzi WW, Missmer SA, Lieberman E, Kajeepeta S, Wall S and Chan GJ (2016) Kangaroo mother care and neonatal outcomes: a meta-analysis. *Pediatrics.* 137(1): 1–16.

Dettwyler K (2013) Full-term Breastfeeding. *AIMS Journal.* 25(3).

West D and Marasco L (2008) *The Breastfeeding Mother's Guide to Making More Milk.* McGraw Hill.

Hazelbaker A (2010) *Tongue-tie: Morphogenesis, Impact, Assessment and Treatment.* Aiden and Eva Press.

Watson-Genna C (2013) *Supporting Sucking Skills in Breastfeeding Infants.* Jones and Bartlett Learning.

Riordan J and Wambach K (2015) *Breastfeeding and Human Lactation.* Enhanced Fifth Edition. Jones and Bartlett Publishers.

Chapter 6

First Steps Nutrition Trust (2019) Infant milks in the UK: A practical guide for health professionals. https://static1.squarespace.com/static/59f75004f09ca48694070f3b/t/5d131024a4f6110001954423/1561530417559/Infant_Milks_June_2019.pdf.

Drudy D, Mullane NR, Quinn T, Wall PG, Fanning S (2006) Enterobacter sakazakii: An Emerging Pathogen in Powdered Infant Formula. *Clinical Infection Diseases*. 42(7): 996–1002.

WHO (1981) *International Code of Marketing of Breast-Milk Substitutes*. Geneva. https://www.who.int/nutrition/publications/infantfeeding/9241562218/en/.

Eglash A, Simon L and The Academy of Breastfeeding Medicine (2017) ABM Clinical Protocol #8: Human Milk Storage Information for Home Use for Full-Term Infants. *Breastfeeding Medicine*. 12(7): 390–95.

NHS (2016) Formula milk: common questions. https://www.nhs.uk/conditions/pregnancy-and-baby/infant-formula-questions/.

First Steps Nutrition Trust (2016) Formula Preparation Machines. https://static1.squarespace.com/static/59f75004f09ca48694070f3b/t/5b2d1f88562fa7f763 3d8bc4/1529683849679/Statement_on_formula_preparation_machines_Nov+2016.pdf.

CHAPTER 7

Duke RE, Bryson S, Hammer LD and Agras WS (2004) The relationship between parental factors at infancy and parent-reported control over children's eating at age 7. *Appetite*. 43(3): 247–52.

Puhl R and Schwartz M (2003) If you are good you can have a cookie: How memories of childhood food rules link to adult eating behaviours. *Eating Behaviours*. 4(3): 283–93.

Brown A (2017) *Why Starting Solids Matters*. Pinter & Martin Ltd.

Du Toit G, Roberts G, Sayre PH, Plaut M, Bahnson HT, Mitchell H and Lack G (2013) Identifying infants at high risk of peanut allergy: the Learning Early About Peanut Allergy (LEAP) screening study. *Journal of Allergy and Clinical Immunology*. 131(1): 135–43.

Perkin MR, Logan K, Marrs T, Radulovic S, Craven J, Flohr C and EAT Study Team (2016) Enquiring about Tolerance (EAT) study: feasibility of an early allergenic food introduction regimen. *Journal of Allergy and Clinical Immunology*. 137(5): 1477–86.

Rapley G (2015) Baby-led weaning: The theory and evidence behind the approach. *Journal of Health Visiting*. 3(3): 144–51.

Garcia AL, Raza S, Parrett A and Wright CM (2013) Nutritional content of infant commercial weaning foods in the UK. *Archives of Disease in Childhood*. 98(10): 793–7.

Rapley G and Murkett T (2008) *Baby-led Weaning: Helping your Baby to Love Good Food*. Random House.

Bonyata K (2018) Is Iron-Supplementation Necessary? https://kellymom.com/nutrition/vitamins/iron/.

Resources

Vanessa Christie

www.vanessachristie.com
Instagram @vanessa_theparentandbabyclinic

General evidence-based guidance on all things breastfeeding, bottle-feeding and giving solids

www.unicef.org.uk/babyfriendly/news-and-research
www.firststepsnutrition.org
www.nice.org.uk
www.who.int
www.ncbi.nlm.nih.gov
www.bfmed.org
www.gpifn.org.uk
https://assets.publishing.service.gov.uk/government/uploads/system/
     uploads/attachment_data/file/725530/SACN_report_on_Feeding_
     in_the_First_Year_of_Life.pdf
www.analyticalarmadillo.co.uk
www.breastfeeding.support

General parenting books

Why Love Matters by Sue Gerhardt
Raising Our Children, Raising Ourselves by Naomi Aldort
Food of Love by Kate Evans
The Life of Dad: The Making of the Modern Father by Dr Anna Machin

General support and information for breastfeeding and bottle-feeding

Lactation Consultants of Great Britain: www.lcgb.org

Association of Breastfeeding Mothers: www.abm.me.uk
The Breastfeeding Network: www.breastfeedingnetwork.org.uk
La Leche League: www.llli.org
The National Childbirth Trust: www.nct.org.uk

Closed Facebook groups for breastfeeding support

Breastfeeding Twins and Triplets UK; UK Relactation and Adoptive
Breastfeeding Support; Inducing Lactation; UK Breastfeeding and
Parenting Support; Breastfeeding Yummy Mummies; Breastfeeding Older
Babies and Beyond; Cow's Milk Protein Allergy in Babies – Support Group
for parents

Breastfeeding helplines
(with trained breastfeeding counsellors)

National Breastfeeding Helpline: 0300 100 0212
The ABM Helpline: 0300 330 5433
The NCT Helpline: 0300 330 0700
The LLL Helpline: 0345 120 2918

Medications and breastfeeding advice and information

UK Drugs in Lactation Advisory Service: www.sps.nhs.uk/ukdilas
The Breastfeeding Network's Drugs in Breast Milk information service:
        druginformation@breastfeedingnetwork.org.uk
Drugs & Lactation database from the US National Library of Medicine:
        www.toxnet.nlm.nih.gov/newtoxnet/lactmed.htm
Medications and Mother's Milk by Thomas Hale

Baby Buddy

Free pregnancy and parenting App from Best Beginnings:
        www.bestbeginnings.org.uk

Breastfeeding aversion

www.breastfeedingaversion.com owned by Zainab Yate

Breastfeeding and your legal rights

www.maternityaction.org.uk

Breast milk and breastfeeding

Milk Matters: Infant Feeding and Immune Disorders by Maureen Minchin

Choking First Aid

'What to do if Your Baby is Choking – First Aid Training – St John Ambulance' www.youtube.com

Crying and Sleepless Children

www.cry-sis.org.uk (national telephone helpline: 0845 122 8669)

Induced lactation

www.asklenore.info/breastfeeding/induced_lactation
Breastfeeding Without Birthing: A Breastfeeding Guide for Mothers through Adoption, Surrogacy, and Other Special Circumstances by Alyssa Schnell
Closed Facebook group: www.facebook.com/groups/inducinglactation

LGBTQIA infant feeding and parenting

https://dianawest.com/lgbtqia-resources/

Mental health and wellbeing

www.pandasfoundation.org.uk
www.mind.org.uk
www.birthtraumaassociation.org.uk
www.traumaticbirthrecovery.com
www.makebirthbetter.org
www.dadsmatteruk.org
www.thenourishapp.com

Milk banking and donor milk

www.heartsmilkbank.org/milk
www.ukamb.org – The UK Association of Milk Banking

Premature and Sick Babies

www.bliss.org

Skin-to-skin and kangaroo care

www.kangaroomothercare.com

Sleep

www.basisonline.org.uk
www.lullabytrust.org.uk
Holistic Sleep Coaching by Lyndsey Hookway (www.feedsleepbond.com)

Tongue-tie

www.tongue-tie.org.uk

Twins & Multiples

www.tamba.org.uk

Vegan and Vegetarian Nutrition

www.vegansociety.com
www.vegsoc.org

Professional Contributors

Nikki Wilson: www.10ofzen.com Instagram/Facebook @tenofzen.
        Facebook Group 'Mindfulness for Mums'
Dr Anna Machin: www.annamachin.com Twitter @dr_aMachin
Nicki Philips: www.niix.fit Instagram/Facebook @niix.fit
Laura Clark: www.lecnutrition.co.uk Instagram/Facebook @lecnutrition
Dr Karen Gurney: www.thehavelockclinic.com Instagram @thesexdoctor
Emma Hayward: www.emmahayward.co.uk
        Instagram @emma_hayward_osteopath

Index

Page numbers in **bold** refer to illustrations

Acknowledgements

It takes a tribe to raise a family and, as I've now discovered, it also takes an extraordinary tribe to write a book.

First and foremost, none of us would be reading this if it weren't for Jonathan Lloyd at Curtis Brown and Jillian Young at Little, Brown, whose belief in me and in my ideas has made writing this book my reality. I will be forever thankful.

To Josephine Dellow for bringing the book to life with her fabulous illustrations and for her never-ending patience with my endless emails. To Jenny Yelverton, whose generosity of time and photography skills have been crazily kind and enormously appreciated. Huge thanks to both of you for sharing my vision. Thank you also to the wonderful women and babies that volunteered their time for the images throughout the book.

My mindfulness teacher, new friend and the beautiful soul that is Nikki Wilson who worked with me to develop Nikki's Zen Zones. Nikki is the founder of 10 of Zen, a social business providing mindfulness tools and training to parents so we can 'stress less and love more'. A proud mum to two small boys, she discovered mindfulness in 2014 to help her navigate her own mental health as a mother. She has developed an online library of free 10-minute meditations tailored to parenthood, runs an online meditation group and teaches wellbeing practitioners how to incorporate 10 of Zen into their work. Thank you Nikki. You are truly an angel.

To all the other professional contributors: Nikki Philips, Dr

Anna Machin, Laura Clark, Emma Hayward and Dr Karen Gurney, a heartfelt thank you for your time, expertise and wisdom.

To all the parents who voluntarily wrote down their thoughts and experiences. It was humbling reading all you had to say. Thank you for your honesty and I wish I could have included all of them!

My family and friends for the time, patience, hugs, meals, drying of tears, endless childcare, cheerleading messages, mountains of clean laundry, proofreading and space you all gave me to write. I am so lucky to have you all in my life.

Amelie and Laria, I am beyond proud of you. Thank you for being so patient with me, knowing when I needed extra kisses and being the hilarious, thoughtful and amazing children you are. And to our newest little lady who is making her entrance to the world within days of finishing this book. I will always treasure this time we've had together with your constant company of wriggles and kicks. Thank you for reminding me when we needed a break. I love all three of you.

And finally, Gav, the one who has lived this with me and has done so with super-human love and understanding. I try to tell you, but it will never be enough, I love you and I promise to never take you for granted, even if you do steal my charger for the rest of my life. You are unquestionably the best husband and dad I could have ever asked for. This book is here because of you.